Pathways
from
Pain
to
Meaning

Translated by Cynthia Hindes

First published in German as *Leben mit dem Schmerz*
by Verlag Freies Geistesleben, Stuttgart in 2009
First published in English in 2024
by Floris Books, Edinburgh

e   Also available as an eBook

British Library CIP available
ISBN 978-178250-920-2

Pathways from Pain to Meaning

*Short Thoughts on Pain in History
and Personal Development*

Iris Paxino

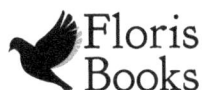
Floris Books

Contents

We are all concerned with living on earth and carrying out the immense task of pouring pain – pouring love – through this star until it becomes transparent, permeated by our spoken and unspoken word – this secret writing with which we make an invisible universe readable for a divine eye.

Nelly Sachs

Introduction:
The Experience of Pain

*Pain is not the truth. Pain is what you have to
go through to find the truth.*

Deepak Chopra, *The Return of Merlin*

There is no one who can say that they have not experienced pain. Our life begins in pain and often ends in it, and in between pain appears in the most varied forms. It seizes us physically, sometimes as a dull warning or as something more sharply expressive; at others it can threaten us almost existentially, completely overwhelming us and breaking us down. And who does not know spiritual pain? The quiet melancholy in which it can sweetly hide, the sadness of the farewell mood that make us wave to the past on the threshold of the future, or the disappointment and resignation that make life taste so bitter? Nor is there any earthly fate that can match the devastating, heartbreaking pain of the loss of a loved one. And how often does the awareness of our own shortcomings – our guilt and failures, our mistakes and omissions – express itself through the pain of realisation?

But what is pain? Why do we refer to the sensation of cutting one's finger in the same way as the mental experience of mortification, despair, loss or homesickness? Can the pain of the exhausted mountain climber be compared to the pain of a woman giving birth? What distinguishes 'pain' from 'hurt'? Is it an indispensable part of being human? And what is it about our experience of pain that can separate us from or connect us to other people?

Generally speaking, pain is an indicator that something is not right with us; it is a sign of injury, disease, or some other disturbance to our well-being. We usually experience it as unpleasant and want to be rid of it as quickly as possible. This desire to be free of pain is common to us all. Through pain, we experience something that should not be the way it is, and it can feel as if the order of our humanity is strangely disturbed.

If we look more closely at pain, we find that it signifies a violation of boundaries, whether physically, such as when we cut ourselves and our skin is broken, or psychologically, such as when a friend says something hurtful and wounds our sense of self. The death of a loved one is also felt as a violation of boundaries: the connection we experienced with another person is destroyed. Pain is thus experienced through the cutting into, or being cut out of, a previously existing unity: be it with oneself, another person or something else besides. Nor does this unity have to be only of a bodily or soul nature. In a spiritual sense, human beings can also feel themselves cut off from a deeper, more meaningful context in their lives.

Yet pain is necessary for human survival. It would be very dangerous for us indeed if, with every contact with the outside world, pain did not remind us of our physical limits. If we were too slow to pull our hand back from a hot stove or too careless with a sharp knife, it would lead to serious, even life-threatening injuries on a daily basis. The absence of pain would mean a lack of self-protection. We can therefore say that pain is also there to keep us safe and free from harm. It serves as a warning signal and can be understood as a sign that something is wrong.

The peculiarity of pain is that it is entirely subjective and personal. Only I can feel my pain; it is not an object of my perception that lies outside of myself. Tissue injuries and the associated irritation of pain receptors or changes to the activity in my brain can be objectively measured, but the experience of pain cannot be quantified. It knows nothing of receptors and nerve impulses; it remains directly connected to my own being. I 'am', in a certain way, my pain. And while I might be able to empathise with another person's suffering, nevertheless I do not experience their pain as though it were my own.

Dealing with pain can vary widely in different instances. The usual approach is to turn our attention towards the pain and work out how to handle it. Bandaging a wound, caring for an injury, and weeping at the grave of a friend who has just died are all forms of giving attention to our pain. We perceive the pain and respond by trying to alleviate it.

But we can also reject and repress pain using the most varied tactics and displacement mechanisms, physical or psychological, and while these procedures represent one way of dealing with the pain, they do not allow us to integrate it.

In daily life we often demonstrate a mix of acceptance and rejection towards pain and suffering. We might be willing to have our aching back treated by physiotherapists, but we do not want to do anything about the emotional suffering that weighs heavily on our shoulders. Or, concerned about cardiac arrhythmia, we might go from doctor to doctor and dutifully take the prescribed medication, but we do not want to confront the pressure of life that we have lived with for years.

Over the course of human history, our relationship to pain has changed. Priests and doctors, healers and shamans, philosophers and scientists, artists and poets have devoted themselves to the questions of how pain arises, what it means, and how it should be dealt with. Human cultures have had, in very different ways, a pain-affirming or pain-rejecting attitude. Pain and suffering have been attributed to various causes and given different meanings. The associations interwoven with pain have changed from culture to culture and from century to century.

From this it is apparent that pain has contributed significantly to the creation of our world as it is today. It has shaped and formed humanity's development. It has accompanied all our wars and served as a tool of oppression. It is present during all periods of transition, from the death throes of the old to the birth pangs of the new, and nothing great has ever been achieved without some degree of deprivation and agony. The overwhelming feeling of being at its mercy and the sense of fate contained in suffering profoundly shape our relationship not just to pain itself, but also to each other and our notions of the divine. It is a primordial phenomenon that takes hold of our whole being and whose appearance is often decisive in our confrontation with ourselves. In this we see pain for what it is and has always been: as an awakening force with the power to raise our consciousness.

Pain in Antiquity: Inseparable from Life

Pain is a great teacher of people. Under its breath, souls unfold.

Marie Freifrau von Ebner-Eschenbach

Pain gives you the right to belong to life.

Otto Roquette

If we look back into human history and consider our changing relationship to pain, we find that people in antiquity had a completely different awareness of life and their own being. In pre-Christian times, they felt themselves to be citizens of the earth while still being united with the world of the gods. They knew that the world of the gods was their true home, and a living spiritual reality permeated everything that surrounded them on earth. In all natural and living phenomena they saw images of divine beings. Matter was not lifeless but rather an expression of living divinity.

Human consciousness during this period was rather dreamy. The alternating states of waking and dreaming were by no means as clearly differentiated as we experience them today, nor were the divine and human realms as sharply separated. Human beings experienced these two worlds as intimately interwoven at all levels of being, just as they experienced the sleeping and daytime worlds as wholly connected.

They also experienced oneness in their bodily and spiritual natures. Their mental states directly determined their physicality, and their physicality was, in turn, an externalised expression of their spiritual nature. In Homer's time, the body's physiognomy was understood as a mirror of the soul. Outer beauty and inner nobility could not be separated; the good always found its expression in beauty. The well-built figures of the Greek heroes were at the same time a reflection of their inner strength and courage. A true hero, full of courage and noble character, could not possibly be outwardly unsightly. Likewise, what was considered ugly was also taken to mean something bad in terms of character. We see from this that the interweaving of the inner and the outer, of human beings and the world, was far more pronounced than we can imagine today.

Human experience, with all its joy and suffering, happiness and pain, was perceived as a gift or punishment from the gods. Human offences, dissipation and disobedience produced pain, and so suffering and illness were believed to be dependent on the way a person lived. But it was still the gods who ruled human destiny. A person's qualities and abilities, how they acted and experienced their fate, were still related to and mediated by the gods at this time. People thus experienced themselves as citizens of a world wherein the gods judged their fate.

The Greeks of early antiquity (around the eighth century BC) did not yet have different terms for external and inner pain. In pre-Homeric times, one does not even find a word for the human body. *Soma* (body) is the word used for a corpse, a lifeless body. There was no expression at that time for the living body. Only the term *demas* (form or gestalt) describes the human being as a unified, living form. The terms *soma* (body), *psyché* (soul) and *nóos* or *nous* (spirit), still known to us today from ancient Greek, were only differentiated in the later centuries of antiquity.

On the trail of pain, we meet a unique figure in Greek mythology who underwent a remarkable transformation due to an incurable, painful wound. It is the centaur Chiron. Chiron's parents were the Titan Kronos and the earthly nymph Philyra. The myth takes us to Thessaly, where Kronos was searching for his newborn son, Zeus. Kronos' wife, Rhea, hid the divine child from his father because she could no longer stand that Kronos always devoured her offspring. During this search, Kronos discovered the beautiful nymph Philyra, who awakened his desire. Afraid, Philyra fled from the unrelenting Titan, transforming herself into a mare to escape his pursuit. Kronos, however, changed himself into a stallion and in this way caught the nymph. Philyra subsequently gave birth to a child, half divine and half animal, who in appearance was half human and half horse: this was the centaur Chiron. But Philyra was terribly frightened when she saw the small, misshapen creature, and begged the gods to transform her into anything else so she would not have to nurse him. Heaven heard her request and transformed her into a linden tree. In this way, Chiron became an orphan.

The legend goes on to relate how Apollo, the god of light, found the abandoned child and took him into his care. He taught Chiron music, poetry, prophecy and healing, and over the years Chiron gained a reputation as a wise teacher and physician. Although physically he resembled the wild and unrestrained centaurs, he was superior to all of them by nature. He was considered a friend of the gods and the wisest and most just of the centaurs. The kings of Greece entrusted their sons to him to instruct them in the arts of life and leadership, and he became the teacher of many famous Greek heroes, such as Jason,

Achilles and Heracles (known by the Romans as Hercules). He also taught Asclepius, the god of healing and the most famous physician of ancient Greece, the secrets of nature and the art of healing.

But Chiron's life took a fateful turn. At a feast of centaurs, who, unlike Chiron, were given to violence after drinking wine, there was a wild brawl. Herakles, who was a guest at this feast, intervened. He shot an arrow with a tip soaked in the poisonous blood of the Hydra and accidentally struck Chiron, who was sitting amid the other centaurs. Deeply upset by the wound he had inflicted on his former teacher, Herakles pulled the arrow out of Chiron's knee. But there was nothing more he could do for him. Although Chiron's half-divine ancestry meant that he did not die from the poison, the wound itself was incurable.

Filled with suffering, Chiron retreated to his cave, where he endured endless torment. He searched tirelessly for herbs to treat his wound, and while he did not find a cure for himself, he gained wisdom in the use of all kinds of medicinal herbs and plants. Through his pain, he also developed a deep compassion for the suffering of others. Whereas his previous life had brought him fame and recognition from all the kings and heroes of Greece, Chiron was no longer sought out by the powerful but by those in pain, and by the sick and the poor. Even though he could not heal himself, he provided help and relief for everyone else. Thus Chiron became known as 'the wounded healer'.

One day, Herakles returned to him. He told Chiron that there was a way to free him from his suffering, but he would have to sacrifice his immortality for another. Herakles further reported that on his long journeys he had met Prometheus, whom Zeus had chained to the Caucasus Mountain as punishment for bringing fire to humanity. Prometheus' liver was eaten by a vulture every day and grew again every night. As the myth says, he had already suffered thirty thousand years of mortal torment.

Shocked by this cruel fate, Herakles asked Zeus to have mercy on Prometheus, but Zeus attached an almost impossible condition for his release. An immortal would have to be found who was willing to renounce his immortality for Prometheus and descend to Hades, the realm of death. Herakles thus went to Chiron with this proposal. Both Chiron and Prometheus had been condemned to live in immense suffering, but if one was prepared to take death upon himself, then the other would be redeemed from his torments.

Chiron, who knew every herb on Earth and yet could find no salvation for himself, was ready to sacrifice his immortality for Prometheus. He died and descended into Hades, the dreaded underworld, where he remained for nine days and nights. But Zeus, moved by Chiron's sacrifice, raised him to heaven as the constellation of the centaur, bestowing immortality upon him once again.

Pain and healing, sacrifice and redemption, life and death, transformation and resurrection all merge in the figure of Chiron. The old world of Titans, cyclopes and centaurs had to give way in the end to the gods of Olympus. A new age was dawning, and with it, a new consciousness. In fulfilling this irreversible change, Chiron, as the teacher of Asclepius, laid the foundations of what would later become European medicine. The healing of our being takes place in the balance between the physical and the soul-spiritual, between the animal and divine aspects of our nature. Chiron's wounded knee points to the connecting link between the middle and the lower human being, where the human ability to straighten up begins and where humans rise up out of the animal realm through their upright posture.

Just as Prometheus, the bringer of fire, stands as a symbol for the human ego, the figure of Chiron anticipates the development of Christian-European humanity. Through suffering and pain, human beings embark on a quest for healing and redemption. On this path, they learn compassion, which enables them to serve and help others. What was once external, fame and recognition of the rich and of kings, is now transformed into a deep inwardness: it becomes the gratitude of the poor and the afflicted. Pain also helps human beings take a further step towards selflessness. For the sake of another, they are prepared to give up even what is most precious to them – in Chiron's case, immortality – and surrender to death. Thus, they attain self-knowledge, compassion and the strength for self-sacrifice through suffering. This means a transformation of their entire being. Only now do they achieve true immortality, not as a birthright, but through their own forces, revealed in the image of Chiron's resurrection in the sky.

Chiron becomes part of a divine world that is renewed through his own doing, through his 'I'. Chiron's pain thus serves as the substance of the transformation.

Let us return to Greek culture and its further dealings with pain. In the fourth century BC, Aristotle organised what was then considered to be current wisdom into ten basic categories. In addition to substance, quantity, quality, relation, place, time, position, state and action, suffering (or passion, from the Greek *paschein*, meaning to suffer or undergo) belonged to the 'primordial substances' of life. Like letters of a heavenly alphabet, these categories were inseparable from the highest reality. Suffering is one of the primal properties of the earthly world, as existential and indispensable to human life as time and space, substance and action.

Accordingly, in ancient Greek culture, the therapeutic treatment of pain consisted not only of physical treatment, it also incorporated a spiritual-philosophical way of life. Pain was not understood as a bodily event but as an imbalance of the entire human being. The medicines administered by Greek physicians were seen by them not merely as plant extracts but as living natural effects and thus actual spiritual forces. Furthermore, only through the control of human passions and the formation of a proper relationship between body and soul could a balance be restored to the human being, which was seen as being ill in its totality.

Well into the transition from Greek to Roman times, pain was understood as a separation from an existing wholeness of the human being. In the second century after Christ, the Greek physician Galen, personal physician to the Roman emperor Marcus Aurelius, described pain as a 'separation of coherence'. For him, even a physical wound was a sensation originating in a separation. The image of a wound as embodied pain and mental pain as a non-material wound encompassed the variation of human suffering. In addition, Galen also described the level of spiritual pain that can arise through the human capacity for consciousness. So we see that European history, from its beginning, viewed pain as having a threefold aspect.

However, the relationship of human beings to the world and thus also to themselves has very much changed in European history since that time. Over the centuries, stronger differentiations have emerged between body and soul, individuals and the world, the human and the divine. Late antiquity and Roman poetry wonderfully demonstrate how the distinction between inside and outside became clearer. A successful commander does not have to possess a beautifully formed exterior outwardly unattractive. Such a notion would have been unimaginable a few centuries earlier. But instead, it is inner values that are important: he must be courageous and have spiritual leadership abilities. Thus we see that physical beauty is no longer a direct mirror of the soul; inner values and outer appearances can even contradict each other. Although the deep feeling for the unity of the human being remained for some epochs, human consciousness was changing, and with it, an ever-more substantial separation between the physical and the soul-spiritual occurred. This change was accompanied by a changed relation of human beings to pain.

Pain and Christianity: Redemption Through Suffering

Only in the tears of pain is the rainbow of a better world reflected.

Christian Friedrich Hebbel

Christianity's history gives a new dimension and meaning to humanity's confrontation with pain. The Christianisation of Europe in the first centuries after Christ was paid for with bloodshed and a unique willingness to endure sacrifice. Pain and punishment, and torture and murder were used as elements of oppression against the small Christian communities, which served only to concentrate the persecuted Christians' will to resist. Overcoming pain through the power of faith and taking upon themselves a martyr's death in veneration of Christ were more potent than the hate-filled attempts to exterminate them.

People of that time experienced a change of consciousness that brought them into a different relationship with the world. They no longer perceived the kingdoms of nature as being interwoven by divine-spiritual entities. The gods gradually withdrew, no longer directing and influencing every step of earthly events, and leaving human beings to stand on their own. Pain, then, became a means of forming a bond between the earthly and the heavenly.

In the origins of Christianity, pain was conceived as the effect of humanity's separation from the divine. At the same time, it was the path to redemption and exaltation. The Bible story tells us how Adam and Eve – that is, 'the human being' – transgressed God's command not to eat from the Tree of Knowledge of Good and Evil. In this way, they detached themselves from the divine bond represented in the image of paradise. However, it is precisely through this detachment that humanity acquired independent consciousness, knowledge and, ultimately, freedom. Pain is therefore the basis and prerequisite for the development of consciousness and human history. It occurs with the expulsion from paradise – that is, with the beginning of human life on earth – and accompanies the development of the earthly world through to its end.

The Christian history of suffering reached its climax and greatest depth in the mystery of Golgotha. By experiencing death on the cross, the Son of God became the bearer of the entire *passio humana*, the entire suffering of humanity. Thus, the possibility of human beings becoming God lies in God becoming human. Suffering and redemption form the bridge between the earthly and the spiritual world. The path of incarnation is already the path of pain, but through suffering and endurance human beings approach spiritual reality in a new, meaningful way.

Only with the end of the world will the history of pain also end. In Revelation it is written: '[God] will wipe every tear from their eyes. There will be no more death or mourning or crying or pain, for the old order of things has passed away' (Rev. 21:4). This is the final word about pain in the Bible, and with it, the arc of human suffering in the Christian tradition ends. And yet a broad span of time filled with pain stretches between these two temporal poles: the beginning and the end of human development.

After the first martyrs, the later saints and monks of the Middle Ages took pain upon themselves in imitation of Christ. The biographical testimonies handed down through the ages are diverse and express both the individual and communal struggle with pain. Persecution and suffering continued to be motifs of Christian history, albeit in the most varied forms. They were seen as a way of honouring God, atoning for sins, or as a test on the way to salvation. Suffering thereby acquired meaning as a transitional stage of development.

Pain also played a central role in the arts, literature and philosophy, producing numerous representations and inter-pretations. Depictions of pain in painting predominantly focused on the crucifixion and placed Christ's suffering at the centre of church art. Matthias Grünewald's Isenheim Altarpiece from the early sixteenth century gives probably the most expressive and harrowing representation of this kind: the image of Christ as the Man of Sorrows in the crucifixion scene. Here, suffering as a sacrifice resulting from a supra-personal loving devotion expressed the deepest and most sublime pain of which a being can be capable. This representation of a pain-filled, deeply human and suffering Christ was initially perceived as a provocation, since it shows the Son of God in his vulnerable humanity. But it is precisely in the experience of pain that the distance between God and humanity is overcome.

The Mother of God immersed in pain under the cross is also portrayed in numerous paintings (for example in Luis de Morales' *Mater Dolorosa*), mostly during the removal of Christ's body from the cross. The uniqueness of the visual expression is poignant in these representations. The meaning of pain has undergone a transformation here – suffering is no longer associated with the principle of punishment or evil, as in early high medieval art, but embodies devotion and sacrificial power.

The previously terrifying nature of pain as punishment now gives way to an empathetic form of expression that focuses on suffering and compassion. Thus the high period of the Passion paintings represents a rich and unique iconography of pain.

The terms for pain also underwent a further differentiation in European culture. Thomas Aquinas distinguished between *dolor*, outer pain, and *tristitia*, sorrow and inner pain. He described the deep devotion of human beings to divine truth as liberation from pain and, at the same time, as an inner healing:

> Therefore, the contemplation of truth alleviates
> affliction or pain, all the more so, the more perfectly
> one has become a lover of truth. Therefore, from
> the contemplation of the Divine ... people feel joy in
> tribulations.[1]

Although pain is still embedded in cosmological–religious contexts, it takes on ever stronger features of individualisation. Human biographies become more individual, and pain is seen as an opportunity for probation and personal development.

In the Christian cultural sphere, we see human beings turning inward. People were thrown into existence more intensely, as Martin Heidegger expressed it a few centuries later in his existential philosophy. As we learned to bear our destiny, the power of endurance as a human virtue acquired a deep meaning for Christian peoples. A life without suffering and pain could hardly be expected, and enduring it became humanity's achievement. The world was increasingly a human one in which individuals suffered war, poverty, hardship and illness. It was also a world in which inner faith in the divine arose as a new strength, replacing the immediate experience of the world of the gods that had been humanity's anchor and support in past ages. Sorrowful events were thus still embedded in a meaning-giving, superordinate whole. What we see happening clearly is the preparation and development of the individual human personality. Pain is one of the formative forces in this process.

3.

Pain in Modern Times:
In Pursuit of a Pain-free Life

*This is my very worst experience: pain makes most people
not great but small.*

Christian Morgenstern

As early as the ninth century, the threefold nature of the human being of body, soul and spirit, which until then had been taken for granted, experienced a decisive rupture. Following the Eighth Ecumenical Council in 869, the Roman Catholic Church abolished the spirit as a component of the human being. Spirit was deemed to be exclusively a component of the divine trinity, meaning the 'Holy Spirit'. What essentially belonged to the divine was denied to human beings. From then on, by decree, humans consisted only of 'body' and 'soul'. The church alone was to decide about the divine-spiritual. This decision would have decisive consequences for the further development of European culture.

The Cartesian separation of body and soul followed a few centuries later. In the emerging dualism of spirit and matter, further fundamental concepts that, in the understanding of earlier times, were perceived as belonging together became detached from each other: body and soul, suffering and meaningfulness. Throughout the sixteenth and seventeenth centuries, authors such as Michel de Montaigne, René Descartes and John Milton largely detached pain from its Christian connections, even as they continued to be influenced by the religiosity of their times. The perception that pain was the expression of a division within the wholeness of the human being was not only increasingly lost but even experienced a meaningful reversal. The experience of pain itself, now increasingly devoid of meaning, was to be separated from the human being altogether.

The progress of the natural sciences, which began in the eighteenth century, gave Western culture an entirely new impetus. The materialism spreading in it brought about a view that reduced the previous understanding of pain. The wholeness of the human being, and pain as a signal of impairment of this wholeness, were no longer included in this modern concept. Pain was only seen as a symptom to be physiologically and experimentally researched, and understood as an affliction to be eliminated. The concept of a physical defect established the idea that pain can be controlled. These developments fuelled an intense polarisation concerning the meaning of the phenomenon of pain. They divided the camps into those who understood pain as an inherently important element of human life and those who doggedly fought it.

In medicine, the production of morphine became the basis for new painkillers, and with the advent of anaesthesia, a veritable era of pain control began. Suffering was increasingly seen as a disorder that should be remedied or eliminated. In 1846, the first tooth extraction under ether occurred in America; this day was celebrated as the 'Death Day of Pain'. One year later, Queen Victoria gave birth to her eighth child under chloroform anaesthesia – birth 'à la reine' became acceptable. America remained the leader in the history of anaesthesiology and, thus, of pain control.

Working in the early twentieth century, the celebrated experimental French surgeon René Leriche declared that pain was not protective, rather it diminished the sufferer, and made them more ill than they would otherwise be. Thus pain begins to be described as not just a symptom but a contributing cause of disease. The understanding of pain as an expression of something important and not merely an eradicable misfortune was largely lost. Questions about the personal meaning of pain thus became silenced, and the destiny of being touched by suffering gave way to the idea of the human being as a functioning machine. Pain and illness were symptoms of a physical defect; they were even devalued as the effects of an unsuccessful adaptation to functional life. Science, through medicine and anaesthesia, and philosophy, through positivism and materialism, found a shared drive in the search for a pain-free life that was as long as possible but perhaps increasingly meaningless.

The campaign against pain and the restriction of suffering were enthusiastically cheered. The only function pain now served was as an indication of a disturbance or disease, and once that task had been fulfilled it could be silenced again. Beyond that, one could live well and gladly without it. It was no longer considered brave to endure pain as it had been in earlier times, since it could be eliminated or avoided. Tolerance of pain decreased, and with it, the ability to live with pain.

But despite the great enthusiasm for progress in pain management, there were staunch critics, even from within scientists' own ranks. French physiologist François Magendie, who himself contributed to research on pain, considered anaesthesia with ether a poison, and compared the anaesthetised patient to a corpse. He insinuated that the practice was more about the surgeon's convenience than the patient's needs, and saw the exposure of the patient while in a state of unconsciousness as degrading.

The German surgeon Johann Friedrich Dieffenbach also complained about the acute separation that anaesthesia brought about between doctor and patient, so that the doctor practices upon the patient while there is no possibility of communication between them. To him, the loss of a personal relationship and interpersonal perception appeared, in essence, as a qualitative decay of the medical healing art.

More clearly heard than the few isolated voices of scientists who were critical of the chemical abolition of pain were the poets and artists of the emerging Romantic and Idealism periods. They considered this biological-mechanical approach too limited, and spoke out against a flattening view of the reality of life. For them, pain was one of the indispensable ingredients in the extraordinary alchemy of life. According to the eighteenth-century poet and philosopher Novalis, 'The new world is born of pain, and in tears the ashes are dissolved into a drink of eternal life.'[2]

Most European philosophers also saw pain as a form-giving, indispensable component of being human. For Immanuel Kant, pain was 'the goad of activity'; only the interplay between pain and pleasure constituted the vitality of life. Johann Gottlieb Fichte likewise saw in pain the impulse to activity, which for us means both joy and pleasure: 'All inertia is overcome by activity.' For Arthur Schopenhauer, pain was an element of the World-Will and an inescapable part of life; knowledge alone created freedom from pain. Friedrich Nietzsche understood pain as a constantly present and formative element shaping life, while Ernst Jünger recognised in it the possibility of self-knowledge and knowledge of the world.

But the philosophical counter-positions, which labelled pain as destruction and disorientation, were also strongly represented. Philosopher and sociologist Helmuth Plessner understood pain as being thrown back on one's body, defenceless, without any possibility of gaining a relationship to it. And it was in this sense that the progress of medicine and pharmacology in the fight against pain continued. A carefree, pain-free life was gradually developing as our society's ideal condition. This was considered as intrinsic as any human right, and the terms 'self-determination' and 'humanity' were defined almost in opposition to the experience of pain. Pain and the resulting impairment of a person's well-being were experienced as a denial of possibilities, and suffering as an externally inflicted evil that had wrongly overtaken them. This injustice of chance had to be eliminated, and so the medically prescribed pain-free life pretended to be a protection against the threat of pain. Suffering was no longer part of being human but damage to a person's well-being that needed to be repaired.

The triumphant march of medical research continued along a seemingly unstoppable path: analgesics were developed, operations were performed under anaesthetic, and at the turn of the nineteenth and twentieth centuries, another medical-pharmacological leap was made. In 1899, Bayer launched aspirin on the market. With it, painkilling tablets were introduced worldwide as 'comfort pills' for everyday use. This represented an immeasurable change to our entire world, and today billions of painkillers are taken each year.

In surgery, the use of narcotics and anaesthesia as the 'technology of numbing pain' opened up many possibilities. The separation of pain conduction pathways made pain completely imperceptible. Human beings who had been separated from their wholeness were now to be separated from the last thing that still reminded them of this wholeness: their pain.

Soon it was not just the suffering patient who forgot that their pain was meant to remind them of something that belonged to them: doctors also lost sight of the wholeness of the sick person. The therapeutic approach no longer applied to the suffering person as a whole but solely to their pain. Just as the trainer was supposed to tame an unpredictable animal, so was the doctor, as a knowledgeable expert, expected to get a grip on pain. The medical healing art lost its skill in recognising and acknowledging human suffering, and with it, the other healing arts also lost their standing. Dealing with pain through empathy and listening, and using herbs, massages, wraps and baths to help people feel and listen to themselves were now scornfully ridiculed and dismissed as unscientific. Healing hands, soothing touch, comforting conversations, and empathic and loving understanding were considered unprofessional. The questions of meaning, context, opportunity and new possibilities through suffering were silenced.

In the twentieth century, the poignant and complex representations of pain in ancient, medieval and early modern art and literature lost their message. Philosophy and religion, deprived of their meaning concerning the existential themes of being, lost their cultural-historical significance. Pain was no longer a reminder of one's wholeness, no longer a sensing of one's limits, and thus a 'boundary experience'. Nor was it a gateway to knowledge or salvation. On the contrary, release from pain was now the only acceptable way to deal with it. All other forms of coping with its occurrence and every attempt to gain something meaningful or positive from it were considered old-fashioned, outdated, unacceptable, even masochistic. The only exceptions were lovesickness, such as heartbreak and the pain of loss. They are still accepted, even sympathetically respected, but are given a place of honour mainly in literature and poetry.

So much for the extreme development of the nineteenth and twentieth centuries in dealing with pain. As a counterbalance, however, it must be said that in earlier times, human consciousness was different and thus people's relationship to pain was different. The living conditions of earlier cultures were also quite different. In past centuries and millennia, people did not live as long. Illnesses ran completely different courses and were often considerably shorter. It may be that acute pain was experienced much more violently, but the many conditions of pain that are part of our time did not exist to this extent in the past. In any case, today's treatment options and life-preserving measures did not exist, and so death was quick to intervene in cases of dramatic wounds, epidemics or other states of illness. People thus experienced pain in a different form than today: though far more exposed to it in acute situations, the constant confrontation with it, for example in long-lasting illnesses or in chronic diseases, did not exist in the same form as today.

Of course, there are states of pain that can leave a person feeling utterly helpless and at the mercy of such terrible agony they feel pushed to the very limit of what they can bear. In this respect, there is much that modern natural science can do to significantly alleviate a person's suffering so that they can regain a certain quality of life. For this, we cannot be thankful enough. This progress gives us a real and decisive opportunity to shape our personal lives.

But progress also brings with it illusions. The opinion that one does not have to put up with pain is ultimately what prompts the consumption of painkillers in such huge quantities, costing millions annually. And yet despite the strong desire to overcome suffering, despite tireless scientific progress and excellent anaesthetics and painkillers, humanity is still far from living a pain-free life. This idealised state has not become a reality, and the vast range of pharmacological products has not yet delivered the final victory.

On the contrary, after the middle of the twentieth century it became increasingly obvious that the triumphal procession against pain could by no means conquer the entire world of human feeling and sensibility. Stubbornly and persistently, the pain that one strictly rejected announced itself again. Chronic pain conditions spread like wildfire, mainly in industrialised nations. From the 1960s and 1970s onwards, pain clinics sprang up like mushrooms after rain. With pain therapy, a special discipline was founded in medicine. Entire psychosomatic departments, pain symposia, medical periodicals and theoretical approaches are now dedicated to therapy-resistant pain. Instead of disappearing from the consciousness of the masses, pain has forced its way to the centre of our attention. It arouses our renewed interest, both personally and socially.

4.

The Language of Pain: The Struggle to Find Expression

Despite all the words of friendship
and gestures of compassion,
every deep pain remains
a hermit on earth.

Nikolaus Lenau

Language, as a mirror of human sensation, creates varied and changing forms of expression for our physical and mental states. Numerous verbs and figurative adjectives express the rich facets of pain. For example, pain can be piercing or cutting, pressing or burning, drilling or biting. There are also many linguistically differentiated descriptions of the sensation of pain in various parts of the body: heads throb, ears ache, legs cramp, lungs burn, hearts are sore. With Paul Valéry, one could say: 'Pain is a very musical matter. One can almost speak about it in musical terms. There are dull and expressive pains, *andante* and *furiosi*, sustained notes, *fermatas* and *arpeggios*, runs – sudden pauses, etc.'

But how does pain 'verbalise itself'? How does it acquire expression and shape? How is it 'heard'? A short linguistic-historical review in German shows us that the word 'suffer' (*leiden*) still meant 'to walk', 'to drive', and 'to be on the way' until the year 860. Today we have completely lost the close connection between suffering (*leide*) and 'leading' (*leiten*), but 'being on the way with suffering' still means, in a certain sense, 'being led through development'.

In German, the word 'pain' (*Schmerz*) is etymologically derived from the Old High German stem *smer-d-*, which means 'to ream', 'to grind', 'to crush'. Originally, in Greek, you can find the word *smerdnos*, which means 'terrible' or 'awful'. In the German-speaking world, the word *smerza* appears for the first time in the year 868. Rhyming with *herza* (meaning 'heart'), it already creates the basis for the genre of heartache poetry from this time forward. Hand in hand with the individual development of consciousness, language development also differentiates the concept of pain more and more finely and subtly in the further course of the Middle Ages.

A remarkable fact is that vowels are more expressive of our inner experiences and personal feelings. Joy, astonishment, pain and disgust are expressed especially by vowels: Aaah! and Oooh!, Ow! and Ew! In contrast, what happens in the world, experienced outside oneself, is predominantly expressed in consonants: rain pattering or dripping, thunder cracking.

The universal character of pain is also shown by the fact that all peoples' physiognomic and physical reactions to it are very similar. In no culture, for example, is hearty laughter associated with pain or a tense contraction of the body understood as joy. The human face conveys to every stranger the clear difference between a joyful and a painful feeling. Acute pain is immediately visible in tense, contracted facial features, which seem to be over-formed or distorted. The suffering person presses their mouth together and pulls their lips inward, even biting them, but when the sensation is too strong to be contained their expression explodes outwards. Edvard Munch's painting *The Scream* exemplifies the inconceivable dimension of inner pain through the figure's wide-open mouth.

Unlike other sensations, such as fear or sadness, pain is not necessarily related to an object, so it cannot always be articulated appropriately. Language may well fail, in which case it is only a cry that corresponds to the immediate experience. At the very least, the sufferer stumbles in their search for an expression that corresponds to their experience. Virginia Woolf describes this struggle of language as follows:

> The merest schoolgirl, when she falls in love, has Shakespeare, Donne, Keats to speak her mind for her; but let a sufferer try to describe a pain in his head to a doctor and language at once runs dry. There is nothing ready made for him. He is forced to coin words himself, and, taking his pain in one hand, and a lump of pure sound in the other (as perhaps the inhabitants of Babel did in the beginning) so to crush them together that a brand-new word in the end drops out. Probably it will be something laughable.[1]

A spasmodic search for words, a spasmodic expression of the human body, are characteristic of acute pain. In chronic suffering, on the other hand, the human face is not tense but rather without tension. It appears depressed and flabby, drooping and altogether shapeless. The posture of the human being also speaks a visible language: the tilted head, stooped sitting, lying hunched, and limp hands. Tears, a universal expression of grief and suffering, are not only an expression but also a 'divestment' of pain.

In either case, the human figure loses the posture that corresponds to it, and the face loses its radiance. In this interweaving between sensation and expression, between body and soul, it becomes clear that the soul's pain is not only experienced but literally 'embodied', just as the body's pain is felt physically and always suffered mentally.

Some cultures train their young people to control their facial features and posture so that pain can be endured 'without batting an eye'. Pain is, therefore, to be managed and controlled. All in all, it can be observed that children are given free rein to react to their pain, whereas adults suppress those reactions much more. So, in every society and in every life, even if culturally and individually very different, there is a certain learning process in dealing with pain. The immediate identification with the sensation of pain can be managed and overcome, at least to a certain degree.

Of course, there are some people who do not feel physical pain at all. As a result of an inherited analgesia, they cannot feel physical pain. The phenomenon of the so-called 'pain artists' is also widely known. The performer who sticks a sword through their tongue or down their throat is a popular sensational moment in many a vaudeville or circus act. Through concentration and intensive mental training, one can learn to focus one's attention and enter an altered state of consciousness in which the sensation of pain is eliminated. People who do not experience pain or can partially master it do exist, but these are rare, exceptional cases.

The rest of us – especially in situations where we are at the mercy of pain – wish we could turn it off completely. At the same time, we are not sufficiently aware that the absence of pain would have disastrous effects on our lives. Painlessness would bring an insensitivity, even numbness, to things and events that would threaten us in real terms. As mentioned in an earlier chapter, we would be highly endangered by ordinary activities if this were so. If, for example, we were engrossed in conversation and were unaware of our hand on the hot stove because we did not feel the pain, the consequences of such a situation could be severe. The burn would still do as much damage to our body as when we were aware of the pain. Leprosy, for example, is a painless disease that is destructive primarily through its numbing effect. The pain receptors on the extremities become numb, causing the sufferers to lose their natural self-protection.

In practical terms, it would also be an overwhelming challenge to show children with no sense of pain the limits of their physical abilities. Pain, at least physical pain, first wants to make us stop and turn back. By feeling pain, greater harm is avoided: pain felt physically becomes pain felt emotionally. The whole person is affected and reacts.

A peculiar aspect of the phenomenon of pain is that, at certain moments, it does not occur as expected. Although the attitude of the natural sciences tends to attribute all processes in the human organism to chemical-physical processes, the occurrence and experience of pain cannot be explained solely by electrophysiological processes in the brain and certain processes in the nervous system. In the case of a severe tissue injury, for example, one would typically also assume a strong experience of pain. But in extreme or highly dramatic shock situations, such as accidents, catastrophes or war, the strongest wounds and injuries are not necessarily experienced immediately, even though the wounded person is conscious. This means that there can be severe tissue damage without pain. In the same way, there can also be severe pain without tissue damage, as in the case of phantom pain, where a part of the body that has been missing for a long time can still be felt as painful.

Therefore, it must be stated that pain is experienced subjectively and individually to the highest degree. The existential threat that we associate with the sensation of pain, or the significance of the experience of pain in the overall context of a situation, is decisive. If a soldier loses a leg in war but is one of only a few to survive, they do not complain superficially about the painful injury but place their loss in the context of the events. This makes it clear that in dealing with pain, our relationship to the world plays a decisive role; it assigns meaning to suffering in the context of our being.

Any physical pain always has a psychological dimension as well. The smallest cut on the finger is always experienced as a feeling. Displeasure and discomfort are at least the weakest emotions of the soul that accompany the feeling of pain. Therefore, it can be said that from the point of view of sensation, all pains are of a mental nature, are mental experiences. The body alone cannot perceive pain. Rather, pain is a sensation of the soul that feels connected to the injured body. Feeling well is also not a purely bodily state but a pleasant way of connecting one's soul to the body.

In medicine over the last two hundred years, pain has been reduced mainly to its signalling function. We expect pain to tell us whether our physical well-being or the integrity of our body is at risk. We call a disease that does not make itself felt at all asymptomatic or sub-clinical. It has not announced itself by the usual harbinger – pain. In our eyes, it is the task of pain to direct our consciousness to an imbalance in our organism.

But to see pain only in its warning character does not do it justice. If it were only a matter of personal well-being, world literature and art would not have reported on it in the most poignant forms, nor would it have shaped the development of the world. Its greatest significance lies in the fact that it belongs to the most elementary of life experiences. It can tear a person away from the world, alienate them from themselves, deprive them of participation in life, and make them lonely and despairing. It is not without reason that pain is feared and experienced as cruel and merciless. When someone has reached their 'pain limit', they know that all differentiated sensations can collapse. In its worst manifestations, pain can cause the world of clear understanding and logical action to sink. Physically, it can bring the sufferer to the brink of death, psychologically, to the limits of madness. Every moment of pain's existence is an entirely immediate and unpredictable new creation.

Therefore, pain is not necessarily a state but rather an event. The sufferer is driven into the borderland experience of the dissolution of the world and its meaning, of being and becoming. Even if the pain does not show itself in this almost annihilating force, a real counterforce is needed to break free from its grip. Consciousness and will are called upon to oppose it. Otherwise, the possibilities of meaningful thinking, feeling and behaviour can hardly be found again.

Taking Rudolf Steiner's description of the twelve senses of the human being, pain belongs, oddly, to the sense of life. With this 'sensory tool', we perceive whether we are hungry or thirsty, whether we are tired or not, whether we are well or not: in short, the state of our being. Pain is, therefore, not an unpleasant, superfluous thing but an extremely central life element. Pain helps us orient ourselves in life and perceive our limits and needs. Without it, courage and daring could not be cultivated; nothing new could be mastered. Through pain, we can 'come to our senses'. At the same time, we experience the deepest layers of our soul through it.

But even if pain can destroy us in its most brutal manifestation, even if we are made to suffer like animals, we are still capable of reflecting on pain and its origin. Only humans can integrate pain into a larger context of life and meaning. Only we humans can wrestle with it, accept it and cope with it. For us, pain always has the character of a challenge: as soon as it is there, something has to be done. It is an experience of self and self-knowledge in the highest degree. It characterises this personal, very individual moment of perceiving and living. Therefore, pain must be understood as a basic human boundary experience with which we must engage. Given its overwhelming presence, it can literally 'leave us speechless' or almost 'slay' us. But pain can also serve us as a language of development or become the language of our own selfhood. Yes, it can help us to first recognise this self so that we encounter ourselves. Pain thus becomes a midwife, helping us to give birth to our own selfhood.

5.

Pain and Consciousness:
Awareness of Our Limitations

Pain is a primordial phenomenon of life.
No higher living being without pain –
but without pain, also no higher life.

Rudolf Frey

The understanding of pain in our time is still strongly influenced by the scientific attitude that all processes of the human organism are chemical-physical. The human soul is not the organ that experiences pleasure and pain; instead, the interaction of molecules, certain processes in the nervous system and the brain, are seen as the cause of the sensation and perception of pain. Over the years, numerous models, concepts and theories about pain and its transmission alternated and contradicted each other until clinical research showed that pain transmission does not work like a simple telegraph system. It is not a one-way street where signals from the body are simply transmitted to the brain but, instead, a highly complex process. Pain is not felt in the brain, as was initially assumed, but at the injured bodily site. However, the person only becomes aware of the sensation when the nerve impulse has reached the brain. Pain is, therefore, a phenomenon of consciousness. Brain processes neither generate nor experience pain; they only make the injury that happened in the body conscious or perceptible.

Our pain inhibition system reacts individually and depending on the situation. This also explains why, for example, pain is perceived in very different ways in the case of severe injuries, shock or emotional arousal. The connection of body and soul (and thus the possibility of self-encounter) and of patient and therapist (of I and Thou) is essential in treating pain. Pain management that focuses only on the disintegrating and splitting-off of pain does not take these connections into account and, for this reason alone, cannot be successful in many cases. These findings make it understandable why some naturopathic treatment methods, which were considered unscientific, and some psychotherapeutic approaches, whose methods were considered ineffective, can nevertheless lead to well-founded success.

The peculiarity of pain is that it binds us physically to the present, mentally to the past, and spiritually to eternity. Physical injury constantly directs our attention to the wound suffered. The sensation of 'being in pain now' is experienced anew in every moment of suffering. Only when the physical sensation of pain has ceased can the person free themselves again from the binding present. Mental pain, on the other hand, directs our gaze to what used to be, what we loved and lost, and lets us live in the memories that constantly surround us. The desire to experience unity with our lost loved one always leads us back into the past and accounts for the quality of this pain.

On the other hand, spiritual pain places before us higher ideals or eternal values that we either cannot satisfy or to which our ordinary reality does not correspond. We suffer from our finiteness, the inadequacy or defectiveness of the individual or the earthly world, which violates the perfection of a higher universe. Whether on the physical, mental or spiritual level, our consciousness is suddenly centred on an area that did not absorb our attention before. Therefore, pain as a phenomenon of consciousness means increased but bound consciousness. This fact is often misjudged in somatically oriented circles. Today's medicine and science assume that the origin and development of other phenomena of consciousness, as with pain, can be explained as arising from the brain. The soul, which is a real and independent entity, the carrier of consciousness and the perception of pain, is not considered on this basis.

However, there are other ways of encountering, understanding and dealing with pain.

6.

Physical Pain:
Illness and Injury

Wounds result in pain, and pain results in people.

Walter Fürst, *Aphoretum*

According to Rudolf Steiner, the human organisation consists of the interaction of several different bodies. There is the physical body, with which we are most familiar. Then there is the etheric body, the first of the supersensible bodies and the bearer of life. The astral body, or soul, is the seat of our consciousness and feelings. Finally, there is our 'I', our individuality. Pain as a phenomenon of consciousness belongs to the astral body and arises when an imbalance occurs between the different bodies of the human being. Steiner said that physical pain can be understood as an intensified consciousness of the body:

> Pain tells us that the astral body is pressing into the
> physical body and the etheric body in an excessive way,
> and acquiring consciousness. Such is pain.[1]

The astral body thus dives too deeply into the physical body and becomes awake there, like a sense organ. Acute physical pain, therefore, means consciousness waking up in the body. The person's attention is continuously directed to the injury. It's as if the astral body is caught in the painful spot and, along with it,

43

almost the entire mental experience of the suffering individual. Even if, for example, only the wrist is broken, the injured person experiences themselves completely within the pain.

It can also be understood why we have the impression that physical pain binds us so strongly to the present, to the currently occurring physical event. The physical body, which is not otherwise perceived in this form, is now experienced forcefully. All other sensory perceptions retreat before the power of this experience. Physical pain thus produces a deepened experience of one's own body. Consciousness, usually asleep for the body, wakes up through pain. In a healthy state, we do not perceive our organs and bones. Only in pain do they become individually noticeable and differentiated. In a way, the intense bodily experience through pain can be seen as an incarnation process in which the soul clings too deeply to the body.

We can explain acute pain in this way. Chronic pain, on the other hand, arises when the astral body clings to the physical body for a more extended period and can no longer free itself.

However, not every physical experience of pain must necessarily result from the astral body encroaching too deeply into the physical organisation. There are also experiences in which, on the contrary, the astral body withdraws from the physical, and a person feels largely detached from their body and what is happening to it. We often encounter this phenomenon, which represents an excarnating process, in cases of abuse or self-injury. It should be noted, however, that this is not only a physical event but also represents psychological trauma. In general, pain perception is far more linked to feelings than is otherwise the case with our usual sensory perception. A purely physical pain without any experiential reference or emotional reaction in an affected person is not possible. Therefore, the phenomenology presented so far can also appear precisely the other way around: an emotional reaction to a traumatic event can also lead to pain. It is therefore crucial to be aware of the fact that the interaction of body and soul is not fixed, but alive and multi-layered.

In a healthy state, consciousness is only mirrored on the body, but in pain, it sinks deeper into the body so that areas of the etheric and physical bodies become too strongly conscious. For this reason, we can also think of pain as 'consciousness in the wrong place'. Since the forces of consciousness are basically transformed life forces, pain is not connected with building up but with processes of breaking down. In a certain respect, these represent forces of death and show themselves, for example, in the form of tissue injuries. To create a renewed equilibrium between the members, it is crucial that the life forces – that is, the etheric body – be strengthened. Rudolf Steiner describes the interaction between soul and body in case of illness as follows:

Normal human life needs the possibility of becoming ill. But there has to be a continuous balance. You see, this allows for the possibility of being able to see a lot in the feeling life of the human being which represents pathological processes, provided we have learnt to see properly. If we are able to observe such things, we can see the approach of an illness a long time before it can be diagnosed physically when the feeling life no longer functions properly. Illness is nothing more than the abnormal feeling life of the human being.

The feeling life remains in the soul element because there is a constant balance in the etheric. As soon as the balance no longer takes place, the feeling life penetrates down into the physical body, combines with the body.

As soon as the feeling life infiltrates the organs, illness appears. So if a person can under normal circumstances maintain his or her feelings in the soul, he or she remains healthy; if he or she cannot do that, the feelings infiltrate down into the organs and illness arises.

I say that by way of introduction so that you can see how important it is for a physician to have a sharp eye also for the human soul life. And basically it is not possible to develop a feeling for diagnosis if we do not have a sharp eye with regard to the soul life.[2]

The stronger and more unbearable the pain is – and thus the deeper the penetration of the astral body – the more completely incapable and helpless we feel: we are all pain. Again, Rudolf Steiner points out that in every pain, both bodily and emotionally, there is an inherent paralysis, which is a sign that the interlocking structure of our being no longer functions in the right way.

In summary, physical pain is an unpleasant sensation of the soul that feels itself bound to the damaged body or injured parts of the body. Correspondingly, in physical well-being, the soul feels connected to the physical in a pleasant way. Suffering and well-being show that the human soul is connected to the whole body. It is by no means identical with it, but it is constantly in interaction with it. A person's consciousness of themselves arises through this mutual interrelation.

Emotional Pain:
Loss and Deprivation

Now you, too, my heart,
have your great lovesickness,
now you, too, are blessed and consecrated
by pain.

Christian Morganstern

Emotional or psychological pain can take many different forms and have many different causes. But in at least one respect it usually has the same feeling quality: an experience of deprivation or loss. Whether a small child is sad to have lost their beloved ball, whether an adolescent in puberty feels lonely and misunderstood, whether a student regrets not having passed an exam, or whether we feel a lack of love or mourn the loss of a beloved partner – all soul pain is about feelings of farewell and loss. According to this, emotional suffering is, in most cases, the pain of deprivation. On the one hand, it is the letting go of what has been, and on the other, the birth of what is coming into being.

The origin of psychological pain shows a different interaction of the elements than with physical pain. Here, the astral body is hindered in appropriately connecting with the etheric body or the physical body. Either the etheric body is in a particularly weakened state and cannot make the right connection with the soul body possible, or it blocks the influence of the astral body because of suffering connected to the experience of loss.

The causes for this can be numerous, but in these occurrences the soul is pushed away from connecting with the organism – or at least with a certain place in the organism. From this, it can be seen phenomenologically that the soul continuously looks to find a particular connection to the body. In sleep it detaches itself, along with the ego, from the physical and etheric bodies, and every morning strives to reconnect itself again with the physical. The natural state of health for the soul is to experience itself in connection with the body.

These interactions also show the contrast between pain and sleep: in sleep, human beings are unconscious because the astral body as the carrier of consciousness has withdrawn. In sleep, a person has no body consciousness at all, only a sleeping soul consciousness. In pain, on the other hand, a person is conscious, they possess a living soul, but they are suffering, which means they also have a living body.

Thus, emotional pain usually indicates that the astral body's connection to the physical and etheric bodies has fallen out of its original equilibrium. The soul has not incarnated deeply enough.

These characterisations only sketchily generalise the relationship of the members to each other based on the phenomenon of pain. To expand on the example of phantom pain given in an earlier chapter, here there is also the pain of loss on the physical level. Similar to the emotional pain of loss, it is a sign of the lack of communication between the astral body and the etheric-physical organisation. Although, for example, an arm has been lost through amputation, the person can still feel pain for a long time at the place where the physical arm used to be. Here, the soul is repeatedly pushed to the place of the former physical limb. The astral body dives into the still-existing life body, but the physical arm is no longer there. The healthy interplay of soul and body is disturbed at this point, and so pain arises.

Pain can be understood in various ways as an expression of an irregular interaction of body and soul. It draws attention to an unhealthy relationship between the various members of a human being. It thus creates the possibility of recognising processes in the organism that would otherwise remain hidden without the pain.

8.

Spiritual Pain:
The Absence of Meaning

All real, great knowledge is born out of pain.

Rudolf Steiner

Spiritual pain goes beyond the bodily and soul levels. It often appears as despair, born of a doubt that has become too strong. It can also be experienced as a loss of meaning or a search for meaning. In any case, it is based on a deep realisation or precisely on the lack of such a realisation. Just as the various forms of emotional pain are facets of an inner experience of deprivation, so is spiritual or mental pain an expression of a profound crisis in cognition.

But what exactly is meant by this? The connection between pain and conscious cognition is described in the story of Adam and Eve, who ate from the Tree of Knowledge and had to experience the pain of expulsion from paradise. Today, we are accustomed to the idea that awareness can lead us past the pain. In other words, it is consciousness or cognition that redeems us from pain.

Throughout human history, it has been known that true knowledge is reached only through pain. According to Rudolf Steiner:

Suffering is a side effect of higher development. We cannot avoid it in attaining insight. Human beings will one day say to themselves: I am grateful for the joy the world gives me, but if I had to face the choice of keeping my joys or my sufferings, I would want to keep my sufferings for the sake of gaining insight. Every suffering presents itself after a certain time as something we cannot do without, because we have to grasp it as part of the development contained within evolution. There is no development without suffering, just as there is no triangle without angles.[1]

The ancient Greeks knew about the connection between suffering and knowledge. The great dramatist Aeschylus wrote, 'He who learns must suffer.'[2] What the great thinkers and philosophers have created, what innumerable artists, discoverers and inventors have also achieved, amount to sublime spiritual records of cognitive pain. All changes in the world have been achieved through pain, and the biographies of those who have advanced humankind are full of sorrow. Every philosophical school gained the knowledge it gave to the world in the shattering pain of existence. In art, Auguste Rodin's *The Thinker* is merely an example of human beings struggling for knowledge, their inner search reflected in the sculpture's physiognomy. Our being is born of knowledge and pain.

One could almost say that in developing the self, human beings have advanced world development over and over again. According to Rudolf Steiner:

Human dignity is increased when what we create is always cruelly destroyed; after all, as a result we must always build and create anew. Our happiness lies in doing and in our accomplishments. Revealed truth is like unearned happiness. Our human dignity depends on our seeking the truth ourselves, guided neither by sensory experience nor by revelation. Once this has been thoroughly recognised, revealed religions will have played themselves out.[3]

And whoever understands this can also understand pain as a path of development that leads to truth and knowledge.

In physical pain, we experience ourselves within the limits of our body. In emotional pain, we relate to our fellow human beings; emotional suffering thus consists of a certain disharmony between ourselves and our surroundings. In spiritual pain, we experience ourselves in relation to the world's superior laws. Suffering on this level consists of a broken harmony between ourselves and creation as such. Steiner also explains:

It is only because we experience self-feeling with self-knowledge, and pleasure and pain with the perception of objects, that we live as individual beings whose existence is not limited to the conceptual relations between us and the rest of the world but who have besides this a special value for ourselves.[4]

The 'I', the Self, the highest entity in human beings, is here the force that speaks out. If we have fallen short of our ideals or have neglected necessary steps of development, we become aware of our failings in relation to a world outside our subjective one. This is where questions concerning meaning begin: a dimension of objectivity opens up in which we experience ourselves as both tool and creator participating in the great world whole.

Thus, our own nature is experienced and recognised through pain. The 'I', the Self, experiences itself in the physical. It experiences both the physical body's limitations and the soul's incapacity. The narrowness of limited ability and the imperfection of our own being lead to the pain of being separated from the 'whole', of being cut off from the divine-cosmic nature of the universe. This is the dimension of the pain of cognition. In this sense, it binds us to eternity through the experience of being insufficiently developed to correspond to the perfection of the whole.

Learning and practising bring us further on this path. Our talents only become abilities when they have gone through practice, meaning also through pain. In this way, new qualities, characteristics and capacities of the outer and inner human being can emerge. Thus, it can be said that pain as a frontier experience in the spiritual realm accompanies the emergence of something new. Overcoming suffering brings about active change and, above all, self-transformation. A new door opens for us and we can step out of our subjectivity and start to see things as they are without us, without our restless wishes, hopes and constant expectations. Being entangled in things, vulnerable on the one hand and unfree on the other, is no longer necessary. The idea that pain gives us gifts may sound strange initially, but it does: it gives us insight and humility. Once we have passed through the eye of the needle through which pain initially squeezes us, a new breadth of understanding and knowledge opens out before us. We learn to see without wanting anything. We learn to understand the world behind the soul. The brightness and darkness, achievements and failures, brokenness and upheavals of our lives become more apparent so that we might confront ourselves and say, 'So this is me.' A personal, very individual moment of perception and suffering arises as self-experience and self-knowledge of the highest degree. It is both a foundational and a boundary experience, an incarnation moment of our Self.

Therefore, 'Know thyself' means also, in the most intrinsic sense, 'Learn through suffering.' The pain leads into the darkness of the ground of existence, in which human beings, thrown back onto the core of their being, can accomplish the reversal into the light of meaningfulness. Thus, the help for any sufferer can be precisely in the experience and the realisation that, 'It is true, it is good, and I accept it because it belongs to me.'

Life means joy and sorrow, but while we happily affirm the joyful we do not gladly embrace the sorrowful, and yet without suffering, life is not whole. For this reason, pain is a wise teacher and a secret friend who faithfully performs its service for us – even if it is never welcome.

Living with Pain:
Understanding its Message

*A healthy person is beautiful, and that occurrence is the ultimate
goal. But a little tiny grain of some disease must come into him
that he also becomes spiritually beautiful.*

Christian Morgenstern

*O Pain,
fill not my mouth with ashes,
now that your fires
have burned my word.*

*My heart,
secretly in league with you,
already senses that pure diamond
you keep hidden
in the bottom of the slag.*

Erika Belte

Diagnosing pain is by no means simple since pain can neither
be measured nor counted according to the classical methods of
scientific medicine. There are costly and complex new methods

by which certain changes in the brain can be detected in connection with pain, but we cannot speak of measuring pain. We only know about it by believing the sufferer's description of their pain. Otherwise, no X-ray, laboratory finding or measuring device can weigh or quantify the pain. Even in cases where pain is feigned, where it is 'simulated', the question arises whether the alleged pain expresses a different kind of psychological distress. Feigned pain is not a logical way of dealing with suffering, but it is at least a distorted attempt to give form to personal suffering. But pain itself is never false; pain is present, whether as an expression of a need in 'another' place (emotional) or as an indication of comprehensible causes (physical). Pain is experienced and is an expression of distress.

The differential diagnostics of pain are not easily manageable, neither for orthodox nor anthroposophical medicine. In anthroposophical medicine, the exact evaluation of the interaction of soul and body – that is the astral body and the etheric-physical body – serves as a basis for this. Methodologically, it can be checked whether the soul has pressed itself too deeply into the body, which results in acute pain, or if the soul body can no longer free itself from the physical body but remains bound there for a longer time, which suggests we are dealing with chronic pain. If, on the other hand, the soul is prevented from rightly connecting with the physical body, one is dealing with the phenomenon of emotional pain. So it is a matter of finding a harmonious equilibrium between the etheric-physical and astral activity.

The correct diagnosis is an absolute prerequisite for the right therapy. Identifying the cause of the pain determines the further course of action and the appropriate treatment steps. In most cases, pain leads the patient to the doctor. Pain also provides information about what is happening in the organism as a whole and what should be uncovered and treated. For the physician, dealing with pain is thus part of almost every patient encounter. Often, it is also the pain and its qualities that sometimes tells the physician more about the nature and biography of their patients than they can do themselves. The therapist needs to show genuine interest, empathy and sensitivity. The therapist's own experiences with pain are also important, as they serve to educate their perceptiveness, compassion and understanding of the patient's own suffering.

Numerous treatments are aimed directly at the pain, initially intensifying it. Other procedures and exercises direct the attention away from the pain, thus creating a balance in the whole organism. Either way, it is essential that therapeutic help not only perceives the material processes of the human body but is aware of the wholeness of the human being and contributes appropriately to an improved balance of the human being's members. Dr Matthias Girke, leader of the Medical Section at the Goetheanum, writes:

> The altered effectiveness of the human being's members leads to therapeutic measures. In case of injury and alteration (e.g. tissue damage) in the area of physical organisation, measures will have to be taken, leading to the re-integration of the disturbed activity of the elements. Accompanying metabolic processes such as inflammation need therapeutic guidance. Appropriate measures must compensate for the pathological 'awakening' of the astral organisation. Finally, it is necessary to support the effectiveness of the ego organization.[1]

As long as medicine is limited to dissolving the symptoms of suffering, we cannot actively shape our own healing. To be able to understand oneself in one's entirety as a suffering person is immanently important. Pain is the indicator that points to where inner and outer tasks are to be taken up. Therefore, a pain therapy that takes into account the various members of the human being includes dealing with all four levels of the human being: first, the perception of the physical conditions of pain and the corresponding treatment; then the strengthening of the etheric body, since it provides the regenerative and healing powers of the organism; then the healing influence on the soul body, since pain as an experience belongs to the astral organisation; and finally, the creation of possibilities for the processing of pain by the ego powers of the patient, since the individuality is the entity that can give meaning to pain and integrate and process it as an experience.

The intensity of the pain plays an essential role. Acute physical pain, in the case of a heart attack or a broken bone, for example, always requires immediate treatment. Making the patient's condition tolerable is of great importance as a first step, for only when the pain becomes bearable will the patient be able to deal with it. The control and relief of pain are necessary components of medical treatment. From a humanistic point of view, however, the question arises as to what significance long-term medicinal pain control has for the relationship between the different members of the human being. Does repressed physical pain become emotional pain? Can a suppressed bodily sensation become mental suffering or depression? Rudolf Steiner presents this connection as follows:

> Of course there are many medicines which provide
> relief. But we have to draw attention to a contradiction

here. External science believes that nothing can be lost. When we rub something, for example, the energy occurs as heat. Something that disappears reappears as a different kind of energy. Analgesics reduce pain and people talk as if the pain had disappeared. Here there is a contradiction with that simple law. When the pain disappears, it reappears somewhere else. We can alleviate as much external pain as we want; it is transformed into soul pain. And people are not aware that these things are connected with the relief of outer pain. This should not prevent us from doing what we think necessary to relieve out pain, but we have to learn to understand the connections and not indulge in illusions in the spiritual field.[2]

Therefore, it should be remembered that treatment is not simply about eliminating pain but also learning to manage it. Medication leads – at least temporarily – to a release from the experience of pain and, thus, to alleviating a patient's suffering. However, painkillers cannot lead to a cure; they merely silence the awareness of the pain at the level experienced. Anyone in the midst of acute pain will empathise with the 'aspirin thinking' of our time. The attempt to end pain as quickly and efficiently as possible is perfectly understandable. However, the way this is done needs to be reconsidered. Is taking medication really about relieving the pain or is it more about masking and suppressing it?

In the case of chronic and emotionally induced pain, painkillers should be considered only as a last resort or given as an adjunct to other therapies. The original form of therapy was the 'laying on of hands'. The soothing 'touch' applied to the suffering person's body and soul alleviated their pain and contributed to their healing. On an emotional level we can say that the 'laying on of hands' involves warm compassion, understanding listening and empathetic consolation. On the spiritual level, the suffering person's encounter with their 'I' and the recognition of its innermost concern is able to help them in their pain. Also, the 'binding', which in the physical sense refers binding the wound, means, in an extended sense of patient care, a real 'bonding' between patient and therapist.

If, in some cases, the experience of pain plays an important part in our development, we might be justified in asking whether automatically administering painkillers is a help or a hindrance. In no way should this be taken to mean that a person should be left in intolerable pain. But some experiences are only possible through pain, and in a society that does everything in its power to abolish it, these experiences can no longer be had in any other way. The so-called 'right to freedom from pain' also means, from a certain point of view, a restriction of the freedom of our experience. Pain demands a confrontation with one's own inner world. As the almost hundred-year-old philosopher Hans-Georg Gadamer recognised and expressed in his last public lecture, suffering leads to an internalisation of life. Thus, it is not a matter of eliminating or abolishing pain, but of understanding and accepting its message. Through this experience we are enabled to develop new, existentially significant insights.

For the therapist, this does not mean taking the pain away from the patient but rendering them able to face their encounter with pain in a way that is suitable for them. In this way, they can also face experiencing their own being and nature. To be 'ready for pain' also means to be 'ready for life'. If you accept the suffering you have experienced, it loses its horror and ferocity. Accepting what is happening is a crucial step in coping with painful experiences. In the therapeutic context, suffering and pain should be understood not as single events but as processes. Their contours and appearances change over time. Everything in life changes: myself, the world around me, my perspective, my desires and needs, my understanding of the world. Changes are inevitable. And so, quite obviously, the perspective from which pain or sorrow was initially viewed will also change. Pain never leaves a person the same as when they encountered it. It transforms them, if they allow it, and therefore it can be said that someone who has suffered has something more to give than they did before. They can also learn to see the possibilities and opportunities ahead of them and not only what they have lost in suffering. Even if, due to loss, the experience of 'less' dominates, so over time, a gain can be experienced, and thus also a new way of 'more'.

One of the most decisive insights in dealing with pain is that suffering itself is merely part of a larger picture, a comprehensive context of meaning. In pain, one is usually blind to the overall picture of one's life situation. Pain can entangle the human spirit in despair, powerlessness or anger. It can become a possession and, in turn, pain can possess a person. They can nurse it, hold on to it, and refuse to give it up. They can also crawl into it or lose themselves in it; they can likewise personify it and fight it as an enemy. Yet it is not only the intensity or force of the pain that determines how a person deals with it or remains at its mercy. If this were the case, then their reaction to pain would be generally predictable. Pain, however, is always an individual experience and involves a very personal way of dealing with it.

Ultimately, we remain free to decide how to relate to our pain. We can choose to search for the meaning in it, and in so doing we are on the way to consciously encountering, understanding, and dealing with it. In dealing with pain, we can become aware of a deeper level of our being. In an entirely new way, we learn to distinguish what is essential from what is non-essential. Pain loses its terror and reveals itself as an instrument of awareness and maturation. We can meet our own higher self, which understands pain as a precious chance for development.

Those who experience meaninglessness in relation to their pain cannot hear the language of their own being, and it is precisely here that we can intervene therapeutically to remove the cloak of incomprehension from their suffering. Through conversation, and with empathy and compassion, the therapist can reach the suffering individual in the loneliness of their pain. They can encourage them to turn to the world with renewed interest, gradually transforming and overcoming the suffering that has marked their inner world. It takes courage to leave the familiar behind – even the familiarity of pain and suffering – and open oneself up to the possibility of new ways of thinking and feeling. It takes an act of will to overcome the pain and create a new image of the future for oneself.

Hermann Hesse writes in his wonderful poem 'Steps': 'A magic dwells in each beginning, / protecting us, telling us how to live.' So also inherent in every pain is a meaning that awakens us and helps us to go on. Indeed, in pain and suffering, there is always a deep meaning that can be discovered through the silence of self-reflection and the humility of self-encounter. Furthermore, with Hesse, we can grasp one of the most decisive qualities of the experience of pain: 'Maybe death's hour too will send us out new-born / towards undreamed lands, / maybe life's call to us will never find an end / Courage my heart, take leave and fare thee well.'[3]

To be open to the future, it is necessary to say farewell to the past. At the threshold of this transition, joy and pain are always very close to each other. If we recognise the positive aspect of the event, we can experience it as enrichment, we can welcome and affirm it. We can then experience this inner process as joy. If we do not immediately see the positive side of the event but first experience the loss, then we feel pain. All of this takes place on the level of the soul. The Self, however, has a completely different criteria for judging pain. It sees pain as a transitional experience on the stony path of development and knows about the potential of these experiences. Indeed, one's higher ego prepares and helps shape these experiences in one's destiny.

To interpret pain as a punishment, as an externally inflicted evil or injustice of fate, merely shows that we are still searching, for whatever way we deal with pain, doubt and struggle are part of it. Body and soul can be deeply hurt and shaken; they can be brutally tormented by suffering and pain and traumatised in the worst way. But our 'I', as a purely spiritual entity, is invulnerable. It knows the service that pain renders us, and can help us to heal.

Returning to the story of Chiron, the wounded healer, we can now see that each one of us is Chiron. Each of us walks a path through wounding and healing to the awakening of the 'I'. Through pain we are led to ourselves and taken beyond ourselves. The descent into pain is fundamentally a process of incarnation. In it, we gain an awareness of the necessity of self-transformation, self-development and sacrificial self-giving. In his book *Philosophy of Existence*, Karl Jaspers elaborates on the sublime insight that one must first become an actual self to become selfless and grow beyond oneself. In accepting our own descent into pain, we achieve the ascent into a new life. Undergoing this process, which is an inner process of death, we recognise the resurrection as an elevation of the soul to the level of the Self. Through this, the transformation of our nature also takes place. Human beings are thus the wounded healers who set out to seek healing for themselves and for the world.

10.

Chronic Pain: The Embodiment of Trauma

Every illness has its own special meaning, for every illness is a purification. One only has to discover from what and for what purpose. There are somewhat reliable conclusions about it, but people prefer to read and think about hundreds and thousands of foreign matters instead of their own. They do not want to learn to read the deep hieroglyphics of their diseases. They are still far more interested ... in the toys of life than in its seriousness – or their own. Herein lies the true incurability of their disease, in their lack of and resistance to knowledge, not in the bacteriological.

Christian Morgenstern

Temporary acute pain, foreseeable in its end, can be experienced with very different qualities, from a slightly unpleasant sensation to an unbearable severity. As a rule, however, acute physical pain does not scar human life. It only seems to interrupt it for a while because our attention is completely focused on it. But it is forgotten again as soon as it is over, at least in most cases. Life goes on without it. However, if the pain takes hold of us and does not let go, if it endures, then the task of dealing with suffering arises.

This kind of pain does not want to give way. It is constantly and brutally present. The analgesic miracle weapons of modern medicine cannot silence it, and a wide variety of different therapeutic approaches have virtually no effect. Those who suffer from chronic pain feel tied to the unpredictable phases in which their pain comes and goes, torn between promising periods of apparent silence and the unfathomable recurrence of their suffering.

But when is pain considered to be chronic?

If length of time is taken as a measure, then we can say that acute pain lasts up to several days, at most several weeks, and rarely several months. Chronic pain, however, is a persistent or recurring pain that lasts six months or longer. A further characteristic of chronic pain is that it usually has significant and long-term effects on the mental state of the one suffering with it.

Worldwide, therapy-resistant pain and chronic diseases have increased markedly in recent decades. Their almost epidemic spread has brought about a decisive rethinking in the theoretical and practical handling of pain. Treating patients with chronic pain has become an important area of medical research and practice. The first specialised pain clinics, where physicians and therapists from different disciplines worked together to treat and alleviate chronic pain, were founded in the 1960s and 1970s. The International Association for the Study of Pain (IASP) was also founded during this time. In the meantime, pain symposia have taken on international dimensions, and periodicals that deal with the topic of pain have become a permanent fixture in medical literature.

Chronic pain also encouraged new approaches to thinking about pain. In 1965, psychologist Ronald Melzack and neuroscientist Patrick Wall proposed their 'gate control' theory of pain, which states that it is the spinal cord that 'decides' whether and how strongly a particular stimulus is experienced as pain. According to Melzack and Wall there is a kind of active input control, which is controlled from the periphery of the body as well as the brain. This helps to explain why our moods can influence our experience of pain, why laughter is sometimes the best medicine and why offering comfort to someone can be more effective than painkillers.[1] The strict separation of body and soul that had characterised the previous scientific approach to pain had to be redefined to make way for new concepts of pain. According to the anthroposophical doctor Markus Treichler:

> Chronic pain, in particular, does not accept the transparent linear cause-and-effect principles; combating it by eliminating it simply does not work here. On the other hand, it has been established that psycho-social factors are decisively involved in the process of pain becoming chronic and that pain experience is shaped to a great extent by personal influences. The highly complex and multi-layered chronic pain process has ultimately led to different combinations of disintegrating and integrating pain treatment approaches. However, they all share one thing: almost all disciplines now understand pain as a 'psycho-physical' unit. Even if the practical handling of this in everyday medical practice still needs improvement, it is at least a standard view today that chronic pain requires an interdisciplinary approach to treatment. According to a classification by the International Society for the Study of Pain, 20% of chronic pain patients have a primary organic cause,

25% have a primary psychogenic cause, and 55% have a psychosomatic cause of pain. This means that only one-fifth of all people suffering from chronic pain have a primary organic cause for their pain. In four-fifths, on the other hand, psychological or psychosomatic causes underlie chronic pain. However, since psychological consequences such as anxiety and depressive disorders are also present in primarily organically caused chronic pain disorders, it is obvious that patients with chronic pain should also always be treated psychiatrically or psychotherapeutically.[2]

It is almost inconceivable that chronically ill people in Germany spend on average seven years going from doctor to doctor and from therapist to therapist until they receive the appropriate psychosomatic diagnosis. Added to this are several hospital visits to clarify the cause of the illness, along with frequently changing drug treatments that do little to reduce their pain and improve their condition. In the same breath, however, it must also be said that very few people are initially prepared to accept that their pain has a psychological component. Most of them deny, at least in the first phase of persistent pain, the possibility that their emotional condition can be expressed in their physical condition. Pain without a clear cause is not an exception in the category of long-lasting physical ailments – quite the contrary. The most frequent headaches are not symptoms of an underlying disease but occur independently. In four out of five cases of back pain, no physical causes can be identified. Contrary to the expectations of most sufferers, the intervertebral disc is the cause of back pain in less than ten per cent of cases. We are therefore dealing with underlying conditions whose causes are often not physically identifiable and are difficult or almost impossible to treat.

In contrast to acute pain, chronic pain no longer appears as a side effect of an illness but develops into an independent condition of its own. The pain shapes the clinical picture so strongly that it is experienced as an illness itself, hence the term 'chronic pain disorder'. The overlapping of physical and emotional events here is striking and expresses the complexity of the pain process in a particularly impressive way. This is the challenge facing pain therapy.

Acute pain indicates a process that is taking place now. Toothache, for example, clearly indicates that a tooth is diseased. A sore throat is inflamed. Acute pains are warning signs or alarm signals indicating a danger or imbalance that usually exists contemporaneously. They have a protective function and trigger purposeful action. The psychological reactions of fright or fear that accompany acute pain are usually temporary and promote goal-directed action. The actions of the affected person or the attending physician normally contribute to alleviating the pain quickly. Even though acute pain can be severe, its cause is usually clear, as is the required treatment. Insofar as an end to the pain is foreseeable, the problem is not experienced as threatening. Even in cases where the immediate future is occupied by pain, such as the result of a bone fracture, the patient can at least rely on the fact that they will return to a pain-free state within a certain period. The patient's orientation within a time-limited framework of pain relief is of great importance for their perception because it serves as motivation and conveys security and confidence.

The situation is different with chronic pain. It, too, indicates that something is wrong, but there is normally no acute danger. Gout patients, for example, understand something is wrong with their musculoskeletal system but, at the same time, know that they are not in immediate danger. They are not concerned with the urgent processes of their body, like someone who treats a wound on their finger. Rather, they are concerned with the pain over the long term. Chronic pain also draws attention to pathological processes, but not primarily as a protective function, as in the case of acute pain. Instead, it points to deeper and more complex processes of the human organism that are not necessarily apparent on the level on which pain is experienced.

There is hardly anyone suffering from chronic pain who does not have their own theory about the origin of their illness. External factors are usually mentioned: cold, humidity, other difficult weather conditions, physical exertion, hard work, the effects of medication. Emotional causes are rarely mentioned, and if at all, then only in passing as merely incidental factors. Certainly, a therapist would not stop at these explanations, recognising that chronic disease is the expression of a much more complex event. But for the person concerned, it is at least an attempt to name a cause for the chronic illness that is comprehensible and gives it meaning. In this way, it becomes possible to deal with the pain and understand it, at least in this first form.

Pain makes people cautious. Whoever suffers from a chronic condition does not think about distant goals and hardly makes any plans. They are grateful for a quiet night or a few hours during the day without this constant companion. The fact that the exact course of their illness is unpredictable makes it particularly insidious, depriving the patient of the prospect of a pain-free future. Exhausted and demoralised, they see no end in sight and lose hope that their condition will ever improve.

For someone suffering with chronic pain, it can so consume their attention that they struggle to carry out ordinary activities. They can no longer relax and the pain disrupts their sleep, which makes everything worse. It distorts their perception of their condition and impacts their emotional state. Unable to stand back from what is happening to them and achieve a more balanced perspective, they are caught in a vicious circle of anger and helplessness. The feeling that they no longer shape their own life and that it is completely dominated and determined by pain can result in severe personality changes, up to and including self-abandonment or aggressive and destructive outbursts. It is well known that depression and chronic pain often occur together, as do an increased potential for addiction and suicidal ideation.

Chronic pain is the expression of an inner event that takes place on another level of the patient's being and becomes embodied as a representation of this event. Somatisation literally means an 'embodiment' of an emotional experience. In this physically experienced form of pain, the affected person does not connect their inner suffering with their mental and emotional states or with stressful life situations; they may even deny they are a factor in anything. They often have a purely somatic understanding of the disease, which does not account for the connection between body and soul. This leads to their inability to relate to the psychic factors contributing to their illness. Or some of them understand the principle of the interplay between soul and body but repress or ignore, to a large extent, the psychological factors at work behind their illness.

Because the pain can become all-consuming, it diminishes the sufferer's capacity for self-awareness. It dominates their mental field, leaving little space for reflecting on what emotional events might lie behind the illness.

Furthermore, sufferers of chronic pain often struggle to express their inner experiences. Representative studies have shown that around twenty per cent of patients in Germany who consult a general practitioner suffer from alexithymia, also known as 'emotional blindness'. This disorder has been recognised only since the middle of the twentieth century and is closely related to the occurrence of chronic diseases. People affected by alexithymia find it difficult to recognise and describe what they are feeling. As a result, their suffering is continually shifted to the physical level, where it is expressed as constant pain. This is then misunderstood as a physical disorder requiring medical treatment.

The chronic ailment is thus to be understood as an unconscious attempt to cope with personal conflict or a biographical crisis that has overwhelmed the soul.

According to Rudolf Steiner, chronic illnesses are brought about when the 'I' or consciousness withdraw to a large extent from events at the inner soul level. In order not to perceive the soul's experience and treat it at the level of the event, the existing problem is shifted to a deeper, even less conscious level through a somatisation process. The 'grievance' thus becomes the 'illness', and the soul's ache becomes a physical affliction.

What do chronic pain sufferers avoid through this alternation of levels of experience? If they were to face the events on the level on which they take place, they might have to experience hurt, sadness, fear, despair or rage. Remorse and blame can also mask themselves as physical illness. Chronic pain tells subtly hidden stories of human biographies for which daytime consciousness finds no words or language. A strong, distressing, shocking or terrible feeling can indeed 'leave us speechless'. We lack the words, not only spoken ones but the ones we need to have an inner conversation with ourselves, with the soul-spiritual parts of ourselves that are capable of coping and dealing with these difficult experiences. If we are unable to process these sensations and experiences, they make their way into the body, where they announce themselves in pain or illness.

In therapeutic work with patients suffering from chronic pain, one often encounters people who have difficulty asserting themselves. They sometimes have an anxious, insecure personality structure and may have difficulty demarcating themselves from others.

Typical consequences of chronic pain are avoidance and protective behaviour, both physical and emotional. The avoidance of painful body postures, the misuse of medications and the reduction of activities to the point of social withdrawal can accompany and aggravate the clinical picture. Avoiding physical activities leads to muscle atrophy through reduced muscular demands, which in turn causes pain-increasing neurophysiological sensitisation processes. In the long run, avoiding social activities leads to isolation, consequently leading to depression. Helplessness, a feeling of powerlessness about their ability to shape their life and a loss of confidence in their own healing powers broadly characterise the chronically ill person's experience of themselves.

Further decisive factors on the patient's side are resignation, pessimistic beliefs, fear of failure and social fears. The tendency to catastrophise ('This pain is killing me!') or become resigned ('Nothing helps anyway! I'm a hopeless case!') unconsciously leads to perpetuating the problem. The trivialisation of the pain experience ('It won't be anything bad!' or 'I'm not going to let the body tell me what to do!') and perseverance strategies ('Pull yourself together!') show patterns of thinking and behaviour that have an impact on the further course of the disease. Fears of social stigma reinforce the patient's anxious expectations. Their intense experience of anxiety and tension generally leads to further intensifying physical symptoms and an inadequate interpretation of the overall situation. It should also be noted that a person's beliefs about their illness can make them extremely resistant to new approaches to dealing with their pain.

The behaviour of the diagnostician also plays a decisive role for the patient. The chosen diagnostic procedures and therapeutic measures, such as X-rays and injection treatments, focus attention – including that of the patient – exclusively on the physical level. The resulting suggestion that the cause of the pain can be found and treated in the body has serious consequences for the chronic pain sufferer. The patient is not encouraged to inquire what it is that their pain is trying to express. On the medical-therapeutic side, the fixation on the bodily level also prevents the inclusion of procedures that consider the mental and emotional aspects of the human being. The patient's family circumstances and professional situation, and the social and emotional stresses of everyday course of the disease.

Today's medical practice is still primarily based on an understanding of disease that adheres to mechanical cause-and-effect principles. Yet the frequently unsuccessful attempts to treat sufferers of chronic pain shows that these approaches are insufficient, perhaps even outdated. Successful pain therapy requires a multidimensional approach and an understanding of the human being in its entirety of body, soul and spirit.

Therapeutic Approaches to Chronic Pain: Gaining Sovereignty

O, pain that first
awakens blind eyes
to see that the world
reflects the I-ness,
that it unseals
our own image, from whose sight
we recoiled.

Erika Beltle

When pain becomes a long-term companion, defying all efforts to treat it, and the prospect of a life without pain seems increasingly remote, then the affected person faces the great challenge of finding a way to manage it. In the context of chronic suffering, it is crucial that the patient gains sovereignty over their pain experience and, step by step, creates new spaces in which to act. What is seemingly unimaginable can be mastered, providing we realise that it is not the pain that is the master of our house but our own Self. For the therapeutic handling of pain, one fact that is of decisive importance is understanding that subjective influences strongly impact the experience and intensity of pain perception. This statement implies that personal experience can be trained and even changed, and that every human being can, in some way, and to a greater or lesser degree, influence the sensation of pain. Even if the pain at times is overwhelming, we still have access to a higher presence, a power that can rise above the suffering and act largely detached from it. Through practising self-encounter and specific therapeutic measures, we can learn to promote and use this precious potential in each of us.

One of the drastic lessons that chronic pain sufferers must learn is that they must not allow themselves to be terrorised by the pain's constant demand to do something. The doing must have a meaningful structure and become purposeful action. Even if the pain cannot be silenced for now, it must first be accepted and embraced. It has become part of the sufferer's life, until they understand how to deal with it better. To 'master' the pain also means to find a way to the 'inner master', to their own Self. This also means establishing a balance between the different members of their being and thus allowing a true healing process to become effective. In the absence, for the time being, of effective treatment, the patient can nevertheless play a crucial and decisive role in dealing with their chronic pain. They can begin to promote and advance their own healing process.

The task of a pain therapist here is to reduce the patient's fear and uncertainty by providing comprehensive information. Furthermore, the therapist should introduce the patient to various possibilities of practising and becoming active, and show them concrete procedures. The patient's experience of pain and their fears about disease need to be taken seriously, and medical therapists must consider that chronic pain can often lead to severe emotional disturbances. On the other hand, it should also be considered that pain is involved in thirty to sixty per cent of mood disorders, especially depression. If the therapist has had to deal with their own pain and they are free of fear in this respect, this can help them build trust with the patient. An empathetic encounter, full of understanding and respect, is the basis for successful joint work.

Pain Management:
A Positive Quality of Life

We cannot withdraw our heart from life, but we can educate
and teach it in such a way that it is superior to chance and can,
unbroken, also watch what is painful.

Hermann Hesse

Behavioural pain treatment is just one of the therapeutic approaches that has proven effective for dealing with permanent pain conditions. This is due to its clear basic principles of problem, goal and action. With the help of pain-management strategies, a transformation of the pain experience can be achieved on various levels. The patient learns relaxation techniques and ways of training their attention that demonstrate how their cognitive, emotional and physical processes can be controlled and influenced. With the help of specific exercises, they can increase their subjective pain threshold and gradually change their attitude towards their pain. This helps them to reduce and even remove the fear they feel with regards to their pain.

To intervene effectively in an event, it is first necessary to have precise knowledge of what is to be influenced. The promotion of self-awareness is therefore an essential first step and component of therapeutic work. Patients suffering with chronic pain often struggle to articulate the qualitatively differentiated characteristics and factors influencing their pain. As a rule, they say that the pain 'appeared quite unexpectedly' and 'for no apparent reason' or 'without anything having happened'. It is difficult for them to give concrete information about cyclical processes or the dynamics of their experience. However, if the therapist asks the patient to describe the course of pain over the last few days, then correlations with certain influencing factors are usually recognisable. The patient can then learn to become aware of these processes and observe them independently.

Perception can be further refined so that certain physical symptoms, for example increased muscle tension, can be felt in a more differentiated way. Through relaxation exercises, it is possible to intervene at this early stage in the development of physical pain. The vicious cycle of pain and tension can be broken.

Attention can also be extended to the emotional and mental levels. Most patients often find that as soon as the sensation of pain occurs, they begin to feel anxious and unsettled: their thoughts become negative, which reinforces the pain. Positive experiences in coping with pain are mostly attributed to others, for example the doctor. But even here, the occurrence of positive and helpful thoughts can help to develop strength and confidence. It is often much easier for us to name what we don't want than what we do – 'I don't want any more pain!' – but here it is crucial for the patient to express what they want in positive terms – 'I want to get healthy!' By defining their goals in this way, the difference between the patient's current situation and the state they hope to achieve can be clarified. This makes the path they need to take much more concrete.

In dealing with chronic pain, it is essential to remember that the patient's perception of it is like a headlight fixed on the sensation and stuck there as if rusted in place. Other stimuli recede into the background and are perceived faintly or even distorted, as if through a veil. Mobility is often limited through the patient restricting their own movement and adopting protective postures, which can lead to further weakening of their muscles. Through step-by-step training, however, limited flexibility can be restored and the patient's mobility can be maintained.

By actively dealing with their suffering in this way, the patient can begin to feel more in control of the healing process. Confidence and a sense of agency are restored. This is why it is crucial for the patient to be actively and consciously involved in the therapeutic process, and not simply to feel as though they are carrying out the doctor's prescriptions.

Finding the courage to enter new therapeutic territory is certainly not easy. It is even more difficult to bring about changes in one's thinking, feeling and activities. Seeing through our personality structures and breaking up ingrained habits is a painful process for anyone, but it is essential in this context. Although this can be especially difficult, it is necessary for the patient to understand the part they may have played in perpetuating their pain without realising it. Often it is the case that other problems in the patient's life have given rise to their condition.

It is even more difficult when the pain is also shown to have a secondary pathogenesis that brings with it certain 'advantages'. For example, the patient's preoccupation with their pain prevents them from dealing with other problems. Then, too, there is the tolerance and leniency, the sympathy and compassion the patient receives from people as a chronically ill person. In the long run, however, every illness becomes a burden for the patient and those around them, and relationships can become severely strained as a result. Nevertheless, the chronic condition can be used, unconsciously, by the patient like a protective shield against certain unpleasant situations or challenges.

Conveying these connections is a challenge for the therapist, one that requires a great deal of compassion and sensitivity. Patients understandably feel aggrieved if they think they are being accused of perpetuating their pain to avoid particular tasks or to manipulate the people around them. In order not to disturb the relationship of trust between therapist and patient, and to avoid misunderstandings at this point, it should be explained in detail that pain disorders are complex and that chronic suffering, in general, can be an expression of mental overwhelm or emotional trauma. It should also be explained that, for many people, pain can take on a helpful function in an unconscious and unnoticed way, such as protecting them from something they are afraid of.

The processes of awareness and change that are demanded of the patient in the therapeutic handling of chronic pain are great. By comparison, chronic pain is familiar and a known quantity, and as difficult as it might be to bear, can be preferable to the unsettling demands of personal change. It is, therefore, crucial that realistic goals are set. The first step is to make the necessary adjustments and take small steps so that the patient can summon up the courage to undergo therapy. In general, there are no standard instruments recommended for chronic diseases, which is why an individually designed therapy is vital. Intensive, step-by-step support from the physician or therapist and transparency in treatment planning significantly contribute to the psychological stabilisation of the patient.

However, despite the many ways of combating pain, there are also pain conditions that defy any treatment. In some cases, all efforts to improve the situation, numerous changes of doctors, therapists and therapies do not lead to relief from the pain. Thrown back on themselves, such patients feel left alone with their pain to deal with it independently. This is where many patients despair, and their doctors and therapists with them. However, if the goal of most pain therapy is to lead a pain-free life again by overcoming it through pain management, the goal in these cases should be to achieve a positive quality of life despite the pain. The task then is for the patient to accept pain as part of their life and to have the courage to live with it by their side. With the help of mental–spiritual exercises, they can adopt a different inner attitude towards their pain. Through greater acceptance they can rise above their suffering, allowing them to retain a sense of agency in their own lives.

13.

Anthroposophic Therapies: Understanding the Whole Human Being

Illness is not suffering. Illness is an opportunity to overcome an obstacle by developing the Christ-power in oneself.

Rudolf Steiner

From the point of view of anthroposophic medicine, chronic pain is a phenomenon that concerns the whole human being. Consequently, an effective pain therapy must start from understanding of the various members of the human being and their relationship to each other. The distinction between the physical, emotional and spiritual dimensions of therapy is of great importance. Undoubtedly, the treatment of pain includes a biological dimension. The administration of medication serves to strengthen the regenerative life forces of the etheric body and exert a healing influence on the human astral organisation to which the pain belongs. Finally, the experience of pain must be processed and understood within the Self of the chronic pain sufferer.

The physician's task is to perceive the patient in the wholeness of their being and to stimulate further treatment according to the configuration of their essential members. It is crucial to involve the patient in the therapeutic process through constant dialogue. After all, they are the one who ultimately carries out the healing process. Even if intensive personal support by the physician or therapist is an indispensable part of the healing process, the purpose of therapy is by no means that the patient must 'endure' or even 'suffer' it. They must participate actively in it and engage with the therapy of their own will.

Chronic pain always tells a very personal story of suffering, so the therapeutic process must be tailored to the individual patient. It is not a unique set of events that make the patient ill, but rather the difficulty they face in coping with them in their individual situation. They need to understand the chronic pain as an unbearable experience of their being that has overtaxed their soul life and ultimately found expression on the physical level in the pain they feel.

The conceptual building blocks of a comprehensive therapy therefore consist of processes of awareness that lead to an understanding of the illness. These are ways of working with mental suffering that offer the patient new and future-oriented perspectives. Emotional development through artistic activity and spiritual training through meditative practice also play a decisive role in this context. The same is true of the trusting relationship that is built up between the patient and therapist and which is the basis of any truly effective therapy. Finally, the patient's growing confidence in their healing powers and the healing process itself provide indispensable positive reinforcement. The developmental steps taken with pain therapy help the patient understand their pain in a new context of meaning.

When used in anthroposophical therapies, eurythmy and rhythmic massage strengthen the etheric body throughout the whole organism and promote the regulation of a renewed balance between the various members. Artistic therapies, such as sculpting, painting, music and speech therapy, create a real and valuable basis for the patient to access their feelings – initially without language or even clear conscious awareness. At the same time, the patient learns to express themselves in an individual and creative way. This non-verbal or preverbal working out of the access to their own deeper experience harmonises the structure of their being. It provides a stable basis for later work on awareness and cognition, which can be carried out as talk therapy, biographical counselling or psychotherapy.

For people in our performance-oriented society, life means activity. Retreat and self-reflection, such as contemplation, meditation, journalling and so on, are often equated with doing nothing and therefore interpreted as a waste of time. In our culture, activities that do not bring any economic benefit have negative connotations. Resigned self-sacrifice or intense activity as a desperate search for redemption from inner pain occur remarkably often in connection with chronic diseases. But these mask the mentally depressed state and can even lead to an 'agitated depression'. In the therapeutic handling of pain, it is important to open connections between soul and body for the patient. The interplay between their emotional pain, arising from want, grievance, conflict and trauma, and the bodily pain of their chronic symptoms should be pointed out to them. In this way, the therapist diverts the patient's attention from their subjective experiences to an objective level that provides them with a greater overview. They are helped to see beyond their despair. The objectivity conveyed, as well as the lawfulness of the overall phenomena, enables the patient to gain a healthy distance from their personal experience of pain. If only mentally at first, they are lifted out of the experience of being subjected to it. At the same time this approach demonstrates to the patient, even if in a different form than they originally assumed, that they are able to act and take charge of their life again.

In a further therapeutic step, an understanding of the patient's psychological history and its connection to biographical development should be established. Past experiences can be viewed and processed, and current events can then be examined against this background. The patient should realise that the pain that plagues them is their own: it is part of what has developed out of the past and directs their attention to very specific themes and motifs in their life. The integration of suffering, the giving of space to pain in their life, is a crucial prerequisite for healing.

It is also therapeutically important to look at the patient's processing and coping abilities and to expand and consolidate them. This includes helping the patient find individual ways of expressing their own being, whose suppressed language has become pain. Two-and-a-half thousand years ago, Hippocrates knew that the first step to healing is contained in the expression of pain: 'What you have words for, you are already over.' Patients should learn to listen to and hear themselves, to express themselves and to converse with themselves. Both dialogue with themselves and conversations with other people (starting with the therapist) are part of developing greater self-awareness, self-confidence and self-expression. These levels need to be enlivened and approached anew so that the patient can find the language to express themselves again, and the organs do not have to express themselves vicariously through pain. Pain merely appears as a signpost.

'Lifting oneself' out of pain also means 'lifting' it from the bodily to the psychological level and encountering it where it originates. It is crucial not only to understand theoretically that pain is part of life but also to identify and accept this pain as our very own. Therefore, healing requires the courage and strength to let the leading soul-spiritual parts of our being come to the fore again. Through them, the unconscious can become conscious, and the emotional trauma that has become a physical illness can be accepted and tackled as a challenge.

Building on these insights and developmental steps, therapy is a matter of working out approaches to solutions together with the patient, from an expanded spiritual perspective to including practising coping strategies. Awareness and spiritual presence – that is, awakening and maintaining the spiritual dimension of the human being in the soul and body – are indispensable prerequisites for progress in the healing process of chronic illnesses. From this point on, it is no longer a question of simply looking for the cause of the pain in the past, but instead working towards development goals and being open to opportunities in the future. The question of where the pain comes from is turned around; instead, the patient asks where it wants to lead them. This change in orientation liberates the patient from what in their past might be keeping them in pain.

Understanding pain as companion that guides the patient on their journey into the future, but then also gratefully releasing it from its role, leads to a real liberation from it. The endurance of pain can, in turn, be overcome by patience and trust. If this succeeds, a process of transformation takes place. The patient is finally able to acknowledge themselves again and understands that the pain is the memory of a forgotten part of their being.

Conclusion:
Pain and Meaning

Suffering is the gateway to love. All the great deeds of sacrificial love would have remained undone had not hardship and suffering called human beings to it.

Luise Rinser

The great questions about the meaning of life, death and pain arise in every philosophy, religion and worldview, and the question of 'why' is associated with every serious experience of pain: 'Why this?' and 'Why me?' There is an immediate association between pain and questions of meaning. It is striking that in almost every biography of an important artist, poet and thinker, pain plays a central and deeply formative role.

Franz Schubert wrote to a friend that it is the works born of one's suffering that give people the greatest pleasure. Johann Sebastian Bach created his most important musical works in old age, when he was almost blind and marked by the death of thirteen of his children. Ludwig van Beethoven was ill, deaf and completely isolated when he composed his ninth symphony, with its incomparably beautiful and powerful 'Ode to Joy'. Music is an art of the heart. All art is a mastery of life. All great composers, poets and painters have articulated their suffering through their artistic creations, condensing the soulful elements of pain into emotional expressions that create a universal world of sounds, colour and language.

Friedrich Schiller was accompanied throughout his life by severe illness and physical pain. Fyodor Dostoevsky wrote his novels between his epileptic crises. Oscar Wilde created his most beautiful poems in prison. Christian Morgenstern, though still very young, spent the last years of his life in sanatoriums with lung disease, hardly able to leave his bed and in the end hardly able to speak. Yet, during these years he produced his most wonderful and precious volumes of poetry.

The world of sculpture and painting also abounds in painful biographies. Living in abject poverty and mental illness, Vincent van Gogh cut off his own ear. He spent his later years in an asylum, struggling with his tortured psyche while also painting some of his most expressive paintings. The Mexican artist Frida Kahlo was seriously injured in a bus accident at eighteen. Her spine was broken in several places, as well as her collarbone, pelvis, leg, foot and several ribs. She spent months in hospital and had to undergo a further thirty operations during her life. She lost several children during pregnancy, had to have several abortions for medical reasons, had several toes amputated and, later, one leg below the knee. She was in constant pain. The traumatic consequences of the accident made her into an artist who transformed her personal life drama into impressive images. Her broken body and lifelong soul pain became carriers of meaning in a transformed, aesthetic form. 'My painting carries the message of pain ... Painting completed my life.'[1] This is how she described and understood herself. She lived and was always wrestling with death, painting while enduring constant pain and fighting against the inexorable deterioration of her body.

Pain thus reveals itself as an existential dimension of development between life and death, between death and its overcoming. Carl Jung gives suffering a central role in human development:

> Without necessity nothing budges, the human personality least of all. It is tremendously conservative, not to say torpid. Only acute necessity is able to rouse it. The developing personality obeys no caprice, no command, no insight, only brute necessity; it needs the motivating force of inner and outer fatalities.[2]

Does this mean suffering and pain are strict educational tools of human destiny? No, not at all, for as Jung also writes: 'The development of personality is a favour that must be paid for dearly.'[3] According to this, pain presents us with a valuable chance to evolve. Whether it can be understood as such, however, depends entirely on the meaning we can derive from it. If no meaning can be discovered in the experience of pain, suffering appears predominantly as a disturbing, even disruptive aspect in the structure of meaning in our experience. In this context, the question arises: how much pain can a person endure or want to endure? A generally valid answer to this question cannot be given, but it can be said that the ability to bear pain is relatively high as long as the pain has a meaningful goal. If, however, this goal is missing, the ability to endure pain decreases considerably.

However, our first reaction to intense pain is not usually to search for its meaning but for its cause, and then for a way to alleviate it. In the case of pain, the path often leads to the doctor, from whom we expect a solution. If such a solution is offered, we consider our search ended. There is no further questioning of what we are suffering from and what the pain wants to tell us; we are just relieved that it has been dealt with. But the absence of pain does not necessarily mean that we have been healed and the cause of pain is not at the same time its meaning. Concerning the cause, we are inclined to accept it as a given, as if it were outside of ourselves. Concerning the meaning, we tend to build up a causal relation – 'It just is' – rather than an intentional one – 'I absolutely want that.' At first we make an attempt to justify pain rather than feeling willingness to take on responsibility for it.

But if the pain remains, the question of what we suffer from also remains. Remarkably, a real answer to this question provides an acceptance of the suffering and, at the same time, great relief, even if the possibility of healing or relief is not immediately given. This is the paradox of pain – that only in pain lies the chance to overcome it! If we only look at the emotional consequences of suffering, then the impression of senselessness prevails. Pain is something that annoys us; illness is something that frightens us; suffering is something that makes us despair. It is only when we place events in a larger context that the meaning of suffering can be revealed, and it is only our active response to suffering, our ability to cope with it, that helps to counteract and even reduce it.

Pain must undoubtedly be treated, but those who define the problem of pain only in these terms and in this way seek to free themselves completely from it are more likely to continue to experience pain. The feeling of helplessness in the face of pain leads the affected person to constantly explain their situation in terms of the past, or to search for what should have happened so that the situation need not have arisen in the first place. By contrast, the more competent a person feels in managing their suffering, the more capable they become in searching for an effective solution. They are consciously able to bring about a change in their existing condition. The perspective of pain is therefore kept within limits through the experience of meaning. It provides a more future-oriented perspective. However, meaning cannot be 'produced', it must be found and lived. The 'will to meaning' means at the same time a 'will to work', and therein also lies hidden the key to one's happiness.

The crucial thing is not just that we suffer, but how we experience it and what we experience through it. Suffering and joy are components of every human life. But whether we are happy or unhappy, whether we experience ourselves as fulfilled or not, depends on how we deal with the circumstances of life. Pain can indeed destroy us, but it can also show us a significant path of development that fills us with gratitude. The realities we experience are always within us, not outside of us. Our soul is the stage upon which our life and experience take place. Our soul is what decides how good or bad we are feeling. Directly linked to it is the meaning we discover in the events of our life.

However, any attempt to artificially give meaning to pain cannot succeed, because meaning cannot be forced. If someone hurts another person, for example, using pain to achieve something specific, then that is about coercion or extortion. They have imposed their will on another person to achieve a certain result. Pain fulfils a purpose but is by no means a life philosophy. Dealing with pain in a masochistic or sadistic way does not allow for the fulfilment of meaning. In instances of self-harm, the body-soul relationship of the person concerned is disturbed. They do not feel their soul sufficiently within their body, as would normally be the case, and need the pain as an amplifier to experience sensation through the body. The person who hurts another and thereby feels satisfaction shows another disturbed relationship to their soul. Only through another's pain can they perceive themselves as a 'master' in their own house. Here, too, the soul needs the pain as a bridge to an understanding of itself, which it otherwise does not have to a sufficient degree.

In both cases, pain is instrumentalised. It serves various selfish purposes and is far from creating meaning.

The most extreme and cruel instrumentalisation of pain is torture. Here it is about using pain to subjugate the individual and dehumanise them using violence. To give pain meaning is to place it into a context that makes it comprehensible and possible to deal with it. The goal of torture, however, is the exact opposite: to bring about a state of helplessness and meaninglessness in the person being tortured. The intention is to traumatise the person's psyche through bodily pain by chaining it so firmly to the body that it negates itself. The pain holds them fast in the agonising present, making impossible any vision of the future where the pain has been comprehended and dealt with. The individual is driven into a borderline experience of the world's dissolution; the Self is supposed to become a non-Self. Thus, the meaning of torture lies precisely in the destruction of meaning.

It is quite risky, even in general terms, to talk about meaning in connection with pain since there is little that calls meaning into question as much as the acute pain of loss or chronic pain. But it is precisely in the most difficult circumstances of human destiny that the great questions of meaning are inextricably linked to suffering: 'Why?', 'What have I done?', 'What is the pain trying to tell me?' From the perspective we have been discussing here, there are no answers to these questions, because they are based on false premises. Pain and suffering are not punishments meted out by angry gods, rather they are general possibilities for us to contemplate ourselves in body, soul and spirit. They are also false in terms of timing, because the question of suffering does not only arise when the disease manifests or when pain first presents itself.

It may seem too simplistic to say that we feel less helpless in the face of a pain we are prepared for than a pain we are not.

But if one recognises that pain is as part of human existence, we can remain calmer about its appearance. An understanding of life that does not repress pain but reckons with it and embraces its possibilities for development prepares us for the fact that experiences such as loss and separation, suffering and pain are part of our existence. The search for meaning in the phenomenon of pain remains directly linked to it. What makes life meaningful and worth living is determined again and again by this life itself. People can learn to appreciate and use the vastness of their experiential worlds by changing their views, goals, perspectives and priorities. This has much to do with maturity and insight, experience and courage in facing one's destiny, and self-knowledge. The sick or mentally injured person's question about the meaning of their life, marked as it is by suffering, is no exception. In this life, too, meaning, or the lack thereof, depends on what that life is lived for and what it is used for. The answer to the question 'Why me?' is therefore: 'Because it is meant for me. It is about me; I am being addressed by destiny.' This can then lead to the question: 'What can I meaningfully do given the present situation?'

A person may complain about the pain that plagues them, but they will no longer complain about the meaninglessness of a life in which pain and illness play a part. They will sooner become a friend of life in all its wondrous manifestations. They will become an understanding companion of the people surrounding them and whom they can assist in need. A wordless understanding of what is happening in the other person will distinguish them. They can think and feel themselves into the most diverse contexts because they are not tugging at life with constant desires and disappointments. It is not the case that suffering corrects a person, but rather that the person can 'correct' their own life through the experience of suffering by overcoming self-absorption. From this perspective of development, pain can be understood not as punishment or denial of possibilities, but as an opportunity.

Rudolf Steiner even goes so far as to say that the fact that pain often seems to outweigh pleasure is 'our *good fortune* as human beings'.[4] Such a thought seems almost absurd to us today since we live in an age that devotes a great deal of scientific research to keeping people as free from pain as possible. And millions of people take painkillers every day because they cannot cope with their pain in any other way. Since pain is a condition of consciousness, the perception of pain decreases as consciousness becomes cloudier; therefore, this approach is initially understandable. Pain should be treated. In the case of a broken leg, it cannot be expected that the patient pull themselves together, get up and simply walk again. Both the treatment of the damaged bone and that of the acute pain are indispensable components of the therapeutic approach. The same is true of mental and emotional pain. Grief and depression must also be treated with medication if the situation demands it. Given the emotional abyss that opens up in a mourner's experience, one cannot demand that they 'pull themselves together' and continue to live their life as before. To be overwhelmed by pain and suffering is, therefore, by no means a goal to strive for in dealing with pain.

But the fact that it is possible in other cultures to alleviate and treat pain largely without medication should make us pause for thought. There are numerous ways to overcome pain. What does our culture have to offer apart from technical and medical developments? What about a return to gentle physical care, to perception and listening, to relaxation and concentration exercises, to consciousness training and meditation?

In the image of the crucifixion as depicted in the Isenheim Altar, we witness the greatest imaginable suffering that culminates in death and, in the image of the resurrection, a liberation from that pain. The agonising and pain-tormented body-consciousness was overcome and redeemed by a spiritually conscious capacity for sacrifice. In the image of Christ, we recognise the willingness to suffer as the transforming power of pain. This Christian path takes humanity's oldest insights further and shows that pain is one of the essential building blocks in the sublime architecture of human biography. According to Steiner it is precisely pain that can lead us to self-knowledge:

> For pain is one of those facts that drive the soul out of the consciousness of its unity with the things of the world ... The fact that events can produce pain in human beings but cannot do so in the external world, however, drives the soul to the recognition of its own special nature. [5]

Experiencing ourselves through pain is, therefore, a step towards self-awareness and self-formation. Pain, as part of the Christian journey, helps us break through the loneliness that always accompanies suffering. As Steiner explains:

> To be separated from what one loves is suffering. But one can be united forever with those whom one loves if the Christ impulse glows through one. One gradually learns to experience this union as a reality.[6]

In this way, an awareness of the other can arise in our hearts. Not only is our loneliness overcome, but we become even more compassionate towards others who are in pain. Compassion is born out of suffering; thus, pain not only transforms us but carries us beyond ourselves. It is one of the great treasures of life not to be abandoned in our suffering. In the sense of the old saying 'A problem shared is a problem halved', through true compassion we can support others and thereby help to make their burden easier to bear. Love, as the basic Christian quality of human existence, does not shy away from the path of pain but understands it as training for selflessness and the transformation of our being.

And there is one last thing that pain can do. When we understand that to be human is to accept that life means change and death means new life, then we can recognise that pain hides the power of knowledge, change and happiness. As free, developing individuals, we can gain the consciousness of spiritual reality through pain. Through this realisation, we can grow beyond our humanity and reach our own divinity as a conscious 'I'.

Seen in this way, pain reveals itself not only as a result of past events, but also as an awakening call from the future. It does not want to destroy us but to shake us awake, because there are things we only understand when we reach a limit. Pain hurts, but we can use it. And even if it appears in such a form that it shatters our expectations and desires, and destroys ideals and everyday reality, we realise it cannot destroy us. For there is in every human being a Self which is peculiar in that it does not belong to itself. It is a Self that can transcend, and only in transcendence find itself.

Endnotes

2. Pain and Christianity: Redemption Through Suffering
1. Aquinas, *Summa Theologica*, Question 38, Article 4.

3. Pain in Modern Times: In Pursuit of a Pain-free Life
1. Novalis, *Henry von Ofterdingen: A Romance*.

4. The Language of Pain: The Struggle to Find Expression
1. Woolf, *On Being Ill*, p. 29.

6. Physical Pain: Illness and Injury
1. Steiner, *Manifestations of Karma*, p. 118.
2. Steiner, *Understanding Healing*, p. 19.

8. Spiritual Pain: The Absence of Meaning
1. Steiner, *The Spiritual Hierarchies and the Physical World*, p. 147.
2. Aeschylus, *Agamemnon*, II.175.
3. Steiner, *Nature's Open Secret*, p. 78.
4. Steiner, *The Philosophy of Freedom*, p. 92.

9. Living with Pain: Understanding its Message
1. Matthias Girke, 'Schmerzverständnis und Schmerztherapie in der Anthroposophischen Medizin' [Understanding of Pain and Pain Therapy in Anthroposophic Medicine], *Der Merkurstab: Zeitschrift für Anthroposophische Medizin*. [The Mercury Staff. Journal of Anthroposophic Medicine] vol. 61, no. 5, Sept/Oct 2008, p. 423.
2. Steiner, *Paths and Goals of the Spiritual Human Being*, p. 33.
3. Hesse, Herman, 'Steps', available at https://www.poetryverse.com/hermann-hesse-poems/steps#:~:text=Steps%20As%20every%20blossom%20fades%20and%20all%20youth,beginning%2C%20pro-tecting%20us%2C%20telling%20us%20how%20to%20live.

10. Chronic Pain: The Embodiment of Trauma

1. Esther Fischer-Homberger, 'Schmerzfreiheit und Schmerzverlust – zur Geschichte des Umgangs mit dem Schmerz [Freedom from Pain and Loss of Pain: On the History of Dealing with Pain]', in *Der chronische Schmerz – eine interdisziplinäre Herausforderung* [Chronic Pain: An Interdisciplinary Challenge], Lorenz Fischer (ed.), Series: 'Complementary Medicine in Interdisciplinary Discourse', vol. 9. Peter Lang, Germany 2006, p. 17.

2. Treichler, Markus, 'Somatoforme Schmerzsyndrome' [Somatoform Pain Syndromes], *Der Merkurstab: Zeitschrift für Anthroposophische Medizin.* [The Mercury Staff. Journal of Anthroposophic Medicine], vol. 61, no. 5, Sept/Oct 2008, p. 459.

Conclusion: Pain and Meaning

1. Herrera Hayden, *Frida Kahlo: Die Gemälde* [Frida Kahlo. Her Paintings], Schirmer/ Mosel, Munich 1992, p. 49.

2. Jung, *The Development of Personality*, p. 173, par. 293.

3. Ibid., par. 294.

4. Steiner, *Nature's Open Secret*, p. 80.

5. Steiner, *The Riddles of Philosophy*, p. 45.

6. Steiner, *Wo und wie findet man den Geist?* [Where and How to Find the Spirit?], p. 379.

Bibliography

Engelhardt, Dietrich von, *Krankheit, Schmerz und Lebenskunst: Eine Kulturgeschichte der Körpererfahrung* [Illness, Pain, and the Art of Living: A Cultural History of Bodily Experience]. Beck Series, vol. 1298, 1999.

Fintelmann, Volker, *Schmerz und Bewusstsein: Wege der Schmerzbewältigung* [Pain and Consciousness: Ways of Coping with Pain]. Gesundheitspflege Initiativ [Healthcare Initiative], Germany 2003.

Fischer, Lorenz (ed.), *Der chronische Schmerz – eine interdisziplinäre Herausforderung* [Chronic Pain – an Interdisciplinary Challenge], Series: Komplementäre Medizin im interdisziplinären Diskurs [Complementary Medicine in Interdisciplinary Discourse], vol. 9, Peter Lang, Germany 2006.

Frankl, Viktor, *Der Mensch vor der Frage nach dem Sinn – Eine Auswahl aus dem Gesamtwerk* [Man and the Question of Meaning – A Selection from the Complete Works], Piper, Germany 1985.

Glier, Barbara, *Chronischen Schmerz bewältigen. Verhaltens-therapeutische Schmerzbehandlung* [Managing Chronic Pain: Behavioral-Therapeutic Treatment of Pain], Pfeiffer bei Klett-Cotta, Germany 2002.

Hayden, Herrera, *Frida Kahlo: Die Gemälde* [Frida Kahlo: Her Paintings], Schirmer/Mosel, Germany 1992.

Jaspers, Karl, *Philosophy of Existence*, University of Pennsylvania Press, USA 1971.

Jung, Carl Gustav, *The Development of Personality* (CW17), Bollingen Series XX, Princeton University Press, USA 1991.

Karger, André and Heinz, Rudolf (eds.), *Trauma und Schmerz: Psychoanalytische, philosophische und sozialwissenschaftliche Perspektiven* [Trauma and Pain: Psychoanalytical, Philosophical and Social-Scientific Perspectives], Edition Psychosozial, Germany 2005.

Lievegoed, Bernard, *Man on the Threshold: Challenge of Inner Development*, Hawthorn Press, UK 1998.

Schönbächler, Georg (ed.), *Schmerz: Perspektiven auf eine menschliche Grunderfahrung* [Pain: Perspectives on a Basic Human Experience], Chronos, Switzerland 2007.

Schneider, Johannes W., *Vom Sinn und Wert der Lebenskrisen. Ein Psychologe zu Problemen des modernen Lebens* [On the Meaning and Value of Life's Crises. A Psychologist on Problems of Modern Life], Verlag am Goetheanum, Switzerland 1998.

Stacher, A. (ed.), *Ganzheitsmedizin und Schmerz* [Holistic Medicine and Pain]. Third Vienna Dialogue. Facultas-Universitätsverlag, Vienna 1993.

Steiner, Rudolf, *Geist und Stoff, Leben und Tod* [Spirit and Matter, Life and Death] (GA66), Dornach 1988.

—, *The Healing Process: Spirit, Nature and Our Bodies* (CW319), SteinerBooks, USA 2010.

—, *Illness and Therapy: Spiritual-Scientific Aspects of Healing* (CW313), Rudolf Steiner Press, UK 2013.

—, *Introducing Anthroposophical Medicine* (CW312), SteinerBooks, USA 2010.

—, *Manifestations of Karma* (CW120), Rudolf Steiner Press, UK 2011.

—, *Nature's Open Secret: Introduction to Goethe's Scientific Writings* (CW1), Anthroposophic Press, USA 2000.

—, *Paths and Goals of the Spiritual Human Being: Life Questions in the Light of Spiritual Science* (CW125), Rudolf Steiner Press, UK 2015.

—, *The Philosophy of Freedom: The Basis for a Modern World Conception* (CW4), Rudolf Steiner Press, UK 2011.

—, *The Riddles of Philosophy* (CW18), Anthroposophic Press, USA 1973.

—, *The Spiritual Hierarchies and the Physical World: Zodiac, Planets and Cosmos* (CW110), Rudolf Steiner Press, UK 2008.

—, *Understanding Healing: Meditative Reflections on Deepening Medicine Through Spiritual Science* (CW316), Rudolf Steiner Press, UK 2014.

—, *Wo und wie findet man den Geist?* [Where and How to Find the Spirit?] (GA57), Dornach 1984.

Weber, Alfons, *Schmerz und Schmerzkrankheiten: Ursachen und Behandlung von akuten und chronischen Schmerzzuständen – Medizinische, psychologische und psychotherapeutische Hilfen* [Pain and Pain Diseases: Causes and Treatment of Acute and Chronic Pain Conditions – Medical, Psychological and Psychotherapeutic Aids], Thieme, Germany 1991.

Woolf, Virginia, *On Being Ill,* Uitgeverij HetMoet, Amsterdam 2021.

Floris Books

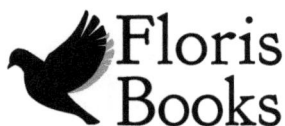

For news on all our **latest books,**
and to receive **exclusive discounts,**
join our mailing list at:

florisbooks.co.uk/signup

Plus subscribers get a FREE book
with every online order!